THE CANCER ANSWER

**Albert Earl Carter
and Larry Lymphocyte**

**A.L.M. Publishers
Scottsdale, Arizona 85260**

Dedication

The *Cancer Answer* is lovingly dedicated to Bonnie, Wendie, Darren, and Melynda: they shared my life with Larry.

Disclaimer

This book is informational only and should not be considered as a substitute for consultation with a duly licensed medical doctor. Any attempt to diagnose and treat an illness should come under the direction of a physician. The author is not a medical doctor and does not purport to offer medical advice, make diagnoses, prescribe remedies for specific medical conditions, or substitute for medical consultation.

When actual persons are referred to herein, the names have been altered and/or initials have been used to protect the privacy of the individuals involved.

TABLE OF CONTENTS

Foreword

IN THE BEGINNING...

Cellular Communication

Don't be surprised if you don't know anything about it. No. I'm not talking about the cellular telephones you've heard about on TV. Not the kind you put in your car, or boat, or airplane. I'm talking about when you really talk to yourself ... and get an answer.

Cellular communication is a lot more advanced than biofeedback. In biofeedback, you're doing all the talking, and your body is doing all the listening. You know your body hears you when it reacts to the commands you give it when you're in the alpha mode. I had a hard time comprehending the principles behind biofeedback when I first heard about it. In fact, I was a very skeptical subject. But it took only one successful session attached to the biofeedback electronic measuring equipment to convince me that I didn't have all the answers. There *is* something to this. It was sort of weird to find out that I really could control my body temperature and the beating of my heart with my thoughts.

I guess that's when I became really interested in my body. I mean, *really* interested. After my experience with biofeedback, the very next day found me in the library searching out all the books I could find on human physiology. Looking back, I guess the librarian must have thought I was a "born-again-reader." I was in that library every second or third day exchanging books.

I became really wrapped up in the way nerve cells transmit electronic messages from one part of the body to another by the use of the smallest amount of electric energy, generated along the cell membrane by the sodium-potassium pump.

At night, I stared at my fingers in fascination as they danced in front of me, doing exactly what I told them to do with a simple thought command. I was communicating. They were reacting. But it wasn't enough.

Finally, one night I connected a pair of wires to an old twelve-volt car battery, added a rheostat so that I could control the amount of electricity, and proceeded to literally shock myself for the next two and one-half hours. I touched my forearm with a bare wire and watched my hand curl into a fist. I found the strategic locations on my thigh that caused my leg to straighten out, and the place on my neck that forced my head to dip forward. Let me tell you, not all of these 'shocking' experiences were pleasant. I found that it took very little electricity to cause the muscles to perform. When I used too much voltage, it hurt. Still, I continued trying to find ways to communicate with *me*.

I'll never forget the exhilaration I felt when Dr. Henry Blaymire, Ph.D., a highly-respected professor of Human Physiology, invited me into his laboratory over at the university. I was there to see one of my very own cells perform on television. I was so excited that I didn't even feel the prick of the needle when the doctor took the blood sample from my ear that he needed to prepare a slide. I do remember that he was very methodical and took the time to explain every step in great detail. But I don't remember what he said.

The microscope was hooked up to a TV monitor. Suddenly, a bit of *me* appeared on television. I saw the round disks of my red blood cells, funny-looking tatters of protein globules, and my white blood cells. My white blood cells caught my attention immediately. They were moving! I had never thought of them *moving* before, but they were moving. They even changed direction, almost as if they knew exactly where they were going.

"Look," Dr. Blaymire said, "watch them phagocytize that piece of dead cell."

"Wow!" I exclaimed. I was truly impressed as the dead matter disappeared. "But why don't they eat the red blood cells?"

"Because the red blood cells belong to the same body. Lymphocytes, the white blood cells, won't eat cells that belong to the same body unless there's something wrong with them," he explained.

"You mean my white blood cells know what to eat and what not to eat?" I asked.

"Yes," the doctor answered. "That little lymphocyte is smarter than you could ever imagine. He even graduated from a school of higher learning called the Thymus before he was allowed to wander around your body like that. He had to learn what he could and could not eat. That's a sensitized T cell. All the cells that go through the Thymus to get their education are called T cells."

That was it. I knew what I had to do. I had to communicate with 'him', or was it 'her'? No, 'him'. Because I am a 'him'. I didn't know how I was going to accomplish this. I just knew I had to. If he was smart enough to graduate from Thymus School and decide what he wanted to eat for lunch, he was also intelligent enough to listen to me.

And *this* is what I'm talking about when I say *cellular communication*. I am talking about the real thing. If you are as successful as I am, you, too, may soon be humming to yourself, "Getting to know you. Getting to know all about you ..."

CHAPTER 1

THE REAL WORLD

Monday: 2:30 p.m.

Mondays are hard for me. In my persona as Professor Albert E. Carter, I teach three physiology classes to students who are not really ready to settle down and endure another week of college work, most likely because Mondays signal an end to a weekend of college fun. But this Monday was especially tough. I had been closeted in my laboratory since the previous Friday afternoon trying to bring the new IBM PC computer I had requested last quarter on-line. Truth to tell, I was no more ready for Monday than any of my students.

I couldn't help reflecting that it was a good thing I had detailed notes on Dr. Bjorn Nordenstrom's book, *Biologically Closed Electric Circuits: Clinical, Experimental, and Theoretical Evidence for an Additional Circulatory System,* in front of me. This book covers two decades of Nordenstrom's important work. His concepts are undeniably fascinating, but potentially revolutionary.

I turned my attention back to what I was saying to my class. ". . . so, when Dr. Nordenstrom measured the electrical

1

properties of the veins, arteries, capillaries, and blood in living animals, he found that the electrical resistance between the blood and walls of the veins and arteries was two-hundred times that of blood itself. In effect, the vessels were acting as insulating cables between the blood flowing through them, the tumor, and the healthy surrounding tissue. When Nordenstrom applied an electric current to the blood vessels, the white blood cells, which carry a negative charge on their surface, were attracted to the positive electrode. Is that clear?

"Speak up. We have time for a few questions before the end of class." I nodded to a studious brunette in the back row. "Erica?"

"Professor Carter, do all unhealthy tissues develop a positive charge?"

"Yes, they do. If the cells of the body are sick and dying, the cell membrane breaks down, thereby producing a positively-charged cellular environment. Blood clots also form in the capillaries as a result of the positive charge. This reduces local circulation and inhibits the spread of infection. Lymphocytes converge on the area from all directions to clean up the mass of dead cells. Anyone else? Yes, Jeff?"

"If all the lymphocytes are attracted to a positive charge, then why don't we just stick a positive electrode into a tumor, turn on the juice, and call the lymphocytes to lunch?"

"You have the right idea, Jeff. Dr. Nordenstrom came to the same conclusions, but we'll have to discuss all that tomorrow. Class dismissed."

As the class stampeded for the door, I brightened. Now, I thought, if I can just get back to my new computer and bring it on-line, I'll be able to explore some of Nordenstrom's ideas for myself. I picked up my notes, shoved them into my brief case, and headed out the door. I was halfway down the hall when I heard a voice hailing me.

"Professor Carter . . . Professor Carter . . ."

Missed it by that much. I sighed and turned back. "Oh,

hi, Mary Jo. Look, I really don't have time to. . ."

"You just don't know how much your class means to me, Professor. I mean, at first, I really didn't like the idea of all those little bugs running around inside me. But when you explained they were killing all the bad ol' germs. . . I mean, I really began to like them. You know, I think I can even feel them runnin' around, 'cause sometimes I feel tingly all over. Especially when you explain them in your class. Do you think. . ."

"Look, Mary Jo, I've got a bunch of them captured in a test tube in my laboratory. They've been in there all weekend. I just have to let them out. Please excuse me."

"Oh my goodness! The poor things. Maybe I could go with you and. . ."

With my most serious frown, I answered, "No, Mary Jo. You might scare them." I think she believed me. I had overheard someone telling her last week that people who bleach their hair too much weaken their eyes, and that's why all blond movie stars wear sunglasses. She had gasped, "Really?" Ever since then, she's been squinting in class. I almost chuckled out loud as I turned away and made my escape.

In the lab, everything was just as I had left it. A mess. Packing boxes tossed in the corner, plastic foam popcorn everywhere. But at least the PC was there waiting to be programmed. If I could just manage to have enough time alone, I would finally be in a position to explore some of Dr. Nordenstrom's theories with the assistance of the computer.

Mercifully, my students are bright and I enjoy my classes, but the week seemed endless. Somehow, I managed to keep interest high in class, and got the job done on the PC as well. I had promised myself a glorious weekend as an investigative detective on the internal workings of the body. And things were shaping up just as I hoped.

Thursday: 7:30 p.m.
Nerve cells transmit electrical messages by alternately

controlling the amount of sodium on the outside surface of the cell membrane, and the amount of potassium on the inside. The sodium-potassium (Na/K) pump pumps three sodium ions out of the cell for every two potassium ions pumped in. Therefore, for every cycle of the pump, the inside of the nerve fiber loses one positive charge. The continuation of this process leads to an excess positive charge on the outside, and an excess negative charge on the inside. Because of the ability of the Na/K pump to create an electrical potential, it's called an electrogenetic pump. Simply stated, all healthy cells of the human body have an electrical charge similar to that of a flashlight battery.

All physiologists understand that. But what Dr. Nordenstrom's work implied was that he had found a way to communicate to the lymphocytes more directly than anyone else had ever been able to do before. And it seemed so simple. Why didn't I think of that? I guess what was really bugging me was that I was afraid someone else was going to be able to control the movement of the lymphocytes before I did. Science is no longer a lifetime labor of love, you know. It's a race. But before I could test out my own theories, I just had to find out if Nordenstrom, the Swedish pioneer, really knew what he was talking about.

I didn't figure I could afford the time it would take to implant cancer tumors inside some lab rats and wait for the ugly buggers to get big enough to poke with electrodes. I didn't want to squander a minute. Besides, I'm not into oncology or cancer research; that's the bailiwick of the guys on the second floor. I'm strictly cells. Healthy cells. More importantly, my cells. All 75 trillion of them. They're the cells I want to communicate with.

It was very exciting to know that Dr. Nordenstrom was killing cancer tumors by connecting a positive wire up to a long needle and poking it into the center of the cancer. All well and very good indeed. He then connected the negative wire up to another long needle and stuck that one into the patient a scant ten inches away from the first electrode. On top of creating an acid in the center of the tumor, the electricity sounded a battle cry that drew white blood cells rushing to the site from various parts of the body. These lymphocytes converged en masse and proceeded to attack the outside of the tumor.

If the U.S. cancer specialists wanted to ignore Nordenstrom's successes, it didn't make any difference to me. The only thing I was interested in finding out was whether I could gather together a congregation of white blood cells large enough to preach to them.

Friday: 9:00 p.m.

I was finally ready to try. My computer was hooked up to an appropriate, highly-sophisticated voltmeter, one capable of measuring very small voltages. I had the negative wire connected to a minute electrode implanted under the skin in my thigh just to the right of my right quadriceps. It was taped down securely. The positive wire was connected to a silver chloride electrode. The oscilloscope was connected in series for recording any and all changes that might (or might not) occur in the electro-potential of my leg.

I felt as if I were wired up and waiting for Dr. Frankenstein to throw the master switch. What some people won't do in the name of science!

I referred to my notes. According to Dr. Nordenstrom's reports, he zapped his patients with between 10 and 20 volts, but that was when he was frying tumors. I wasn't interested in electrocuting tumors. All I wanted to know was how much energy was needed to call the lymphocytes to dinner. Back to the notes again. This is no time to make a mistake. Okay, the electrical potential inside a nerve at rest is -90 millivolts. When a nerve gets excited, it can change its electrical field to +35 millivolts in one ten-thousandth of a second. I decided that it was safe enough to start with one-quarter of a volt.

After carefully swabbing the left side of my right thigh with alcohol, I inserted the cathode under the skin (ouch) and taped it down. It hurt a little, but no more than being poked in the eye with a sharp stick. I then studied all of my equipment, closely scanning all the dials. It was a "go." I took a deep breath and flipped the switch. Lights blinked on. I looked over all the instruments again, looking for the off-light that should be on, or the blinking-light that shouldn't be blinking. Everything was as it should be.

I felt nothing. Thirty seconds went by. I checked my pulse and my body temperature. Both normal. I turned on the electronic stethoscope and put on the earphones. The continuous sound of 'flub-dub flub-dub' indicated that my heart was bored by the whole procedure.

An hour went by. In spite of the electricity being fed into my leg, I still felt nothing, except disappointment. I turned up the volume of the stethoscope until I could hear the blood whooshing through the arteries in my legs. I agreed with my heart. This was boring. I moved the business end of the stethoscope over my abdomen. As a youth, I was embarrassed when my hungry stomach growled loud enough to be heard by someone else. Wow! Even though I hadn't eaten for hours, the workings of my apparently still very busy digestive tract sounded like a sausage factory in full production. The thought was mildly entertaining, but I was still bored.

Most scientific research consists of a flash of inspiration, setting up an experiment to test out a theory, and a lot of waiting. I edged the volume up higher and counseled myself to patience. I was listening to the blood coursing through my right thigh when I first heard it.

"Can . . . you . . . hear . . . me?" The voice was tiny and strange, but very distinct.

I must be picking up a radio transmission from across the campus, I thought to myself.

"No . . . Professor. I'm . . . talking . . . to . . . you."

Now, that's impressive, I thought. These communication students must be into mind reading.

"Telepathic . . . communication . . . isn't . . . hard," the little voice responded to my unspoken thought. "Anybody . . . can . . . do . . . it . . . with . . . practice. But . . . this . . . isn't . . . a . . . telepathic communication. Don't . . . move . . . your . . . stethoscope."

Suddenly the experiment didn't seem important any longer. I began trying to figure out logically how I could be receiving a radio transmission. And, wonder of wonders, how my very thoughts were being transmitted. I looked down. The head of the stethoscope was resting on my thigh, touching the silver chloride electrode. Ah, that's it. That must be what's picking up my thought patterns. The stethoscope is touching the silver electrode.

You're . . . getting . . . close, . . . Professor . . . Carter. But . . . That's . . . not . . . it."

I turned up the volume of the stethoscope still further.

"Thank you," said the voice. "This is going to be easier than you thought."

Okay, I'll play. I sent more thoughts to 'them.' Congratulations, whoever you are. This is a great demonstration of some very impressive technology. But *who* are you, and *where* are you?

"I am known to you as a lymphocyte, one of many."

"You're pulling my leg!" I blurted out loud.

"That would be quite impossible, because of my size. But I'm just below the silver chloride electrode in your leg. By the way, would you please turn down the energy? It's getting crowded in here."

I looked down at my thigh and saw it was red. Wow, I thought to myself, it really works! My thigh is inflamed. I must have brought together a whole congregation of lymphocytes. I . . .

"Now that you have our attention, what is it you want to

say?" asked the voice.

"I don't know," I stammered aloud. "I didn't expect to get this far when I was mapping out the project. You're an unexpected development."

"In that case, Professor Carter, I have something to say to you."

"You what?"

"I've been trying to get through to you for a long time."

I don't believe this, I thought to myself. Cells can't talk.

"I'm not talking, Carter. I'm communicating. All the cells of your body communicate. We do it all the time. When you stub your toe on the edge of the couch, how do you think the cells of your toe tell the cells of your brain that the big toe on your right foot hurts? If we didn't communicate, you wouldn't know when to say 'ouch.' And when you're trying to thread a needle, the cells of your eyes have to communicate with your finger cells or the thread couldn't possibly slip smoothly through that little eye of the needle."

"Yes, of course. But those are messages sent by the nerve cells." I argued.

"You're right, Professor Carter. But, during any form of communication, there must be a sender *and* a receiver."

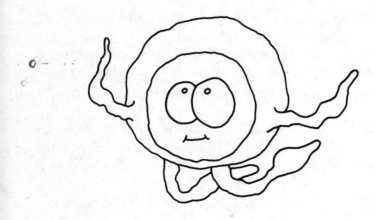

This is silly, I thought. Here I am in the middle of the night arguing with myself. I must be going crazy.

"Not at all, Carter. You just need a little more understanding. You have simply been underestimating your ability to communicate with your own body. But I don't have time to argue. I'm a very busy cell, you know. However, I do have plenty of time to teach."

In answer, I sent the thought: All right. What do you need?

"I need you to write a book. You see, I can't type."

Bibliography

DiPolo, R and Beauge, L: The Calcium Pump and Sodium-Calcium Exchange in Squid Axons. Annu Rev Physiol., 45:313, 1983.

Hodgkin, AL, and Huxley, AF: Quantitative Description of Membrane Current and Its Application to Conduction and Excitation in Nerve. J Physiol, London: 117:500, 1952.

Taubes, G: An Electrifying Possibility. Discover Magazine, April 1986.

CHAPTER 2

COMMUNICATING

One of the problems every author faces is how to write nonfiction that is at once educational *and* interesting. Those of us who write in the medical field are further hampered by the need to use the precise medical terminology of the scientific world to insure accuracy. This difficulty has limited most readers of medical material to their fellow men and women of science who can easily decipher the terminology. What this means is that, while our scientists are totally enthralled with the complex intrigue going on inside our bodies at any given moment, they find they have trouble reaching an audience because of the difficulty in communicating with the rest of us. Those among us who understand the big scientific terms already know the story. Those among us who don't know the story are befuddled by the scientific jargon and lose interest.

I am in the unique position of being able to fabricate a story designed with the non-scientific reader in mind. In this way, I can help you comprehend, at least in part, the miraculous and almost incredible variety of activities that are going on inside you at any given moment just to keep you alive. This book is based on a true story. The names and faces have been changed to protect you from boredom.

Hey, that's not all that bad, I thought as I read over the opening paragraphs of this chapter.

"I'm glad you approve, Carter," the small now-familiar voice said. "Keep typing, and try to clear your mind of any extraneous thoughts."

Now, I don't know about you, but I have a hard time taking suggestions from my wife without other thoughts creeping in, let alone from a tiny amoeba floating around someplace inside of me. In fact, this relationship I have somehow developed with one of my cells was forced on me. I want you to know that right from the start.

During that long night in the laboratory when I had first heard the voice, I found I could get rid of it by moving the stethoscope away from the electrode in my leg. That worked . . . for about ten minutes. I had removed the measuring devices, stuck Band-Aids™ on the two incisions in my thigh, and was limping toward the door when I noticed a buzzing inside my head. At first I thought it was the overhead lights, but the sound continued after I flipped off the switch. Shaking my head and tapping the side of it with the heel of my hand like a swimmer with water in his ear hadn't worked either. Then the buzz deep inside my right ear had gradually turned into faint but distinct words. The voice came slowly at first.

"Can . . . you . . . hear . . . me?"

I tried to ignore it.

"Do . . . you . . . understand?"

I must be going bonkers, I thought.

"Oh, good," the voice said with satisfaction. "You do hear me. I need you to write a book."

"About what?"

"Us. You and us. All of us."

"Us?"

"Yes. All the cells of your body."

"But there are already lots of books about cells written by great scientists. They know all about cells."

"Look, Carter, I don't want to disillusion you. But if what you've been reading lately is everything the scientists and medical men know about the cells of your body, then they need this book as much as anyone."

"How do you know what I've been reading?"

"Everything you experience, including everything you read, is indelibly recorded inside the DNA of the cells of your body. Where do you think your memory is anyway?"

"In my brain."

"Your scientists haven't found it."

"My brain?"

"No. Your memory. As a matter of fact, each of your senses has its own memory."

"You mean that each of my five senses has a memory of its own?" I asked.

"Each of your more than *thirteen* different senses has its own memory. Read your own scientific literature. It will tell you."

"All right, but how do you know what I read?"

"What do you do when you want to learn more about a subject?"

"I go to the library and research it."

"Exactly. Just as all the books in all the libraries of the world are available to you for your edification, so, too, all the experiences of your life are available to us."

"Are you telling me that everything I've ever read is available to you right now?"

"Certainly. How else can you explain the principles of hypnotism? Under hypnosis, the subject can recall a long-forgotten experience in exact detail. Do you remember reading the Nancy Drew and Hardy Boys mysteries in your teens?"

"Yes."

"So do I."

"I never thought of a cell having a memory."

"I know."

"Okay. I hear you. I either have to accept you, or admit I'm going crazy. Either way, I'm going to have a hard time explaining you."

"You won't have to. . . until our book is published. You see, I expect you to list me as co-author."

Friday: 3:20 p.m.

After dismissing the students in my last class, I was free for the weekend. I couldn't wait to get into the project. I sat down at my word processor, placed my fingers on the home keys, and cleared my mind. I couldn't believe I was actually awaiting dictation from a bit of protoplasm floating around somewhere inside me. If nothing else, this should prove interesting.

"All right, little voice," I said aloud. "Speak to me. I'll type. Nobody will ever believe this, but then, neither do I."

"Wait until you read what you've typed," I heard.

"Where should we begin then?"

"Let's try the beginning."

This is what I typed:

The basic unit of life is the cell. Almost all living things, whether plants or animals, are made up of cells. Some minute forms of life consist of a single cell. Larger forms of life are built of many cells.

Life for all of us began the same way. You were a single cell once. The vital genetic information from your mother's side of the family was present in the nucleus of the egg that was to become you. When it was united with the genetic information in the sperm of your father, the new you began to grow. Immediately after conception, the single cell that signals the beginning of a new life begins to divide and multiply. In a process known to science as *mitosis,* a single cell divides to become two - but it doesn't actually cut itself in half. Instead,

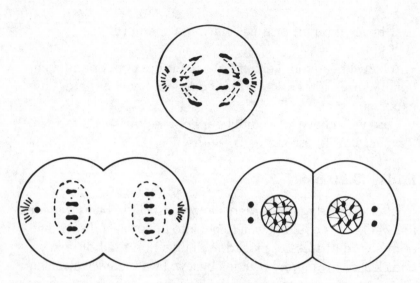

the bundle of chromosomes present in the cell first converges in the exact center, and then separates into two identical bundles of genes. Each bundle of chromosomal programming then migrates to opposite poles. At this point, the single cell looks rather like the figure eight. When what the scientists call cell *division* is complete, the single cell has miraculously *multiplied* itself into two exact duplicates.

What you *are* is governed primarily by the cells of your embryo. By the time you burrowed into your mother's uterus, just days after being conceived, you had become 32 cells strong. Your scientists call you a *trophoblast*. Although they are few in number, your cells have already arranged themselves in an outer layer surrounding a central cell mass. Cellular communication is vital. In accordance with their strict instructions, the cells set themselves in place to become the inner, middle, and outer tissues of your body.

The complete and perfect development of your body requires the interaction of three processes. Your cells must understand and exactly execute: *differentiation*, *morphogenesis*, and *growth*. These processes might be likened to a kind of animated jigsaw puzzle. Each individual cell precisely identifies its appropriate neighborhood and becomes acquainted with those who live next door. Working together, they progressively assemble into tissues and organs. Indelibly recorded in the deoxyribonucleic acid (more familiarly known as the DNA) of each cell is the original genetic programming which does not vary from the original single cell. But each cell also carries the dramatically different instructions each separate family of cells will follow. The programming of each cell teaches it how it is supposed to function in concert with its neighbor, as well as what information it will send and receive.

Differentiation is the genetic information which directs all the cells in the tiny embryo to diversify and transform themselves into the more than two hundred cell types that make up the various muscles, cartilage, bones, nervous system, immune system, eyes, and other tissues of your adult body.

Morphogenesis, or spatial organization, is the programming which determines that a certain family of identical types of cells evolves, for example, into a hand, instead of a foot. Without morphogenesis instruction, you might be born with two left hands, or hands where your feet should be, and vice versa.

Growth instruction governs the size of the adult body. It is the growth law programming which insures that your cells know when to stop multiplying, so that your body reaches its proper size at the proper time and then stops growing.

"Wait a minute," I said. "How does a cell know what it's supposed to do?" I wanted to test his knowledge and I was tired of typing anyway.

"Don't stop now, Carter. I'm on a roll here. Keep typing."

I sighed, but complied:

All cells have the same DNA, the blueprint of your finished body. Once a cell knows its location, it reads only the part of the DNA that informs it of its responsibility. The rest of the information imprinted in the DNA master plan is turned off permanently.

Maybe this will make it easier to understand. Imagine that all the cells in the body are humans seated in the central section of a huge football stadium. Each human is occupying his assigned seat in his assigned row. Let's say that this group of humans is part of the half-time program. Each one has a large card with one color on one side, and a different color on the other, plus written instructions telling him exactly what to do at what time during the show. On certain signals, all the humans hold up their large cards. If they have read their location instruction properly, and are in the right seat in the right row, and if they hold up the right side of the card, they will spell out a message.

Every cell has its own address also. The cells of the index finger have a specific location, and so do the cells of the thumb. Your left arm and right arm, for example, developed completely independently from tiny millimeter-long buds of tissue on opposite sides of you as an embryo, yet they end up of equal length.

"But how did all the cells get an exact copy of the blueprint of my body?"

"Type, Carter. Go with the flow, human. Stop interrupting."

At the moment of conception when the egg and sperm joined, the master plan for your body was established in that one cell. When it divided, it passed the blueprint on to its daughter cells. When those two cells divided, each one passed the blueprint on to two more daughter cells, and then you were four. Each cell is exactly alike and each one is just as intelligent as the other. Each cell reproduces the blueprint exactly, and each cell divides again and again and again. Eventually, each of the 75 trillion cells that comprise your adult body contains the same blueprint established at the moment you were conceived.

"That's amazing!" I said aloud. "It's only been in the last twenty-five years that our scientists have identified the blueprint of the cell as DNA. The combination of complexity and exactness of the DNA is akin to the complexity of the whole universe, and even more fascinating."

"I'm glad you're beginning to appreciate us, Carter. Your health, indeed your very life, depends on the health and life of your cells."

"And almost everyone knows that the genes in the DNA control heredity, traits passed on from the parent to the child," I interjected.

"True. But what most people don't realize is that those same genes control the day-to-day functioning of the cells, as well as our reproduction."

"Okay. The genes control cell function by determining what substances will be synthesized within each cell . . . what structures, what enzymes, what chemicals."

"Right, *Professor* Carter. But you're the student now and I'm the teacher. Who's writing this book anyway?"

"If you want to get technical, I am."

"It was my idea."

"A cell can't have 'ideas.' You're simply reading *my* ideas and putting them into your words. No, my words."

"We're not going to get anywhere if you keep arguing with yourself like this."

"When you're right, you're right," I agreed. "Please continue."

"Here goes. Start typing:"

Indelibly recorded in the DNA of each cell is how to produce every protein molecule your body will ever need. We cells also carry programming on how to digest various foods, how you see, how to produce red blood cells, the hair on your head, even the fingernails on your fingers. The information and instruction in the DNA is so exact that the tiny bones in your right little finger are a mirror image of the tiny bones in your left little finger, even though the cells on opposite sides of your body have never been properly introduced.

"I'm impressed. Dr. Carl Sagan says that if all the information recorded in just one DNA molecule could be translated into the English language and then printed in books, it would take a huge library to hold the complete set. Dr. Sagan figures it would work out to around four thousand books, each one the size of the Bible," I added.

"Who's this Sagan guy, Carter?"

"Dr. Sagan has done a lot of important research on the origin of life in earth's primeval environment," I explained. "In fact, he's probably one of the greatest scientists of our time."

"I see. Well, even at that, I think he's underestimated our full intelligence. But, as you pointed out, Carter, Dr. Sagan could only have known about our cellular DNA library for the last twenty-five years."

"Don't blame him. We humans had to wait for the advent of the microscope before we could even begin to study the various parts of you cells, you know. Long before we knew anything about what was inside the nucleus, we discovered that all animal and human cells appeared to have three main parts: the cell membrane, the cytoplasm, and the nucleus.

"Our scientists found out that the cell membrane is the outside surface of the cell and is composed of protein and fat. We call it the lipo-protein barrier. The *cytoplasm, protoplasm,* or intracellular fluid, are tucked neatly inside the membrane. These are scientific terms we use interchangeably to describe the water inside the cell. We determined that this colorless fluid holds millions of other tiny and very intricate cell parts."

"Good, Carter! You're not such a bad writer yourself."

"Thanks," I said shortly. "I guess you'll have to admit that we humans aren't as dumb as you thought."

"Not quite. Still, even with your electronic microscopes, your scientists are just barely scratching the surface of the vast quantity of knowledge locked up in each cell."

"We'll get there." I fired another question at him. "How long do cells live?"

"Do you want to continue bickering, Carter? Or shall we get on with it?"

"Let's get on with it. I'm ready. Go!"

I believe your question was: 'How long do cells live?' That depends on how you define life. Most cells don't 'die' in the way that humans think of death. Some cells, including blood cells, live less than a month. But some of the nerve cells, including all your brain cells, live your entire life. But remember, when one of us cells divides, two new cells start life afresh. Instead of aging and dying, each old cell becomes two new, vibrant young cells. On the whole, by the end of each year, your body is composed of new cells. What this means is that every year you have almost a completely new body. And you don't even have to retrain it, because the intelligence has been passed on to all those new cells. When you're fully grown, cell division slows somewhat and you begin to age. New cells continue to replace old and worn-out cells, but more slowly the older you get.

"You're just full of information, aren't you?"

"More than you think" he quipped. "Keep working, Carter."

Each type of cell is specifically adapted to perform one or more particular function. For example, your red blood cells, 25 trillion in all, transport oxygen from the lungs to the tissues, and carbon dioxide from the tissues back to the lungs. You expel poisonous carbon dioxide every time you exhale. Some cells have the ability to contract; these are the muscle cells. Other cells are sensitive to light and form the *retina* of the eye. Still other cells are clear. They form the *cornea*, the lens of the eye, and allow light to pass through to the retina. Bone cells have the ability to absorb minerals and deposit them around the outside of their membrane. Other cells produce hormones. Still others are responsible for producing the thousands of different proteins your body needs from the 22 amino acids available for the construction of all cells and the intelligent management of your entire body.

"Hold on here. You haven't mentioned lymphocytes."

"I'm an intelligent and very well organized cell, Carter. Trust me. We have a whole chapter coming up on the entire immune system. We'll get to it in due time. Just keep on typing."

So you see, although the many cells of your body look and act differently, all of us have certain basic characteristics. Contrary to popular *human* opinion, Carter, all cells require the same nutrients. All cells require what your scientists call *glucose,* or blood sugar. We all require certain amino acids, vitamins, minerals, and enzymes. And all cells use oxygen to burn fuel. We give off carbon dioxide and metabolic wastes, which are delivered to the fluids surrounding us as end products of various chemical reactions.

"Okay. Let's see if I've got it. What you're telling me is that my body is actually a city of cells, a civilized social order of about 75 trillion cells, all precisely organized into different functional structures. Some of these structured families of cells are called organs, bones, tissues, and so on. Each functional structure has to contribute its share to the maintenance of my exact internal environment, what the medical men call *homeostasis.*"

"Homeostasis, schomeostasis. Whatever you humans want to call it is fine with me. You *are* beginning to see the big picture, Carter. But there's more:"

You humans live in a gaseous environment composed primarily of oxygen and nitrogen. You call it air. But we cells live internally in a watery environment known as extracellular fluid. Just as long as normal conditions are maintained in your internal environment, the cells of your body will continue to live and function properly. Each cell benefits from the correct chemical balance of your body, what you call homeostasis. But, in turn, each cell contributes its share toward the maintenance of homeostasis. This reciprocal interplay provides a continuous automaticity of your body, unless the cells of one or more functional system lose their ability to contribute their share to normal functioning. When this happens, all of the cells suffer. Moderate dysfunction of a family of cells leads to illness, but extreme dysfunction of any of the important families of cells leads to death.

"Are you saying that the definition of any illness is the moderate dysfunction of certain cells when they fail to do their part?"

"Yes."

"Does this mean that all our doctors really need to do is identify the cells that aren't doing their part and call them to repentance?"

"I see you're beginning to understand the importance of the book already."

"You make it sound so simple."

"On the contrary, Carter. But let's get this down on paper:"

The functions we cells perform to keep you alive are incredibly complex. All you have to do is live. We've been doing our jobs for thousands of years, yet your best scientists admit that they are only now beginning to understand our work. Just wait until you find out what we're going to write about cancer!

"I can hardly wait," I said. "Keep going. I'll keep typing:"

If there is an insufficiency of some types of cells within your body, these cells will grow and reproduce themselves very rapidly until appropriate numbers of them are again available. For instance, did you know that as much as seven-eighths of your liver can be removed surgically? The cells present in the remaining one-eighth portion of your liver will grow and divide again and again until your liver mass returns almost to normal size.

"You're kidding! Is that true?"

"Of course. I told you cells are supremely intelligent. Besides the liver, additional cell families have the same ability:"

The same effect occurs within almost all glandular cell families, the cells of bone marrow, subcutaneous tissue, the intestinal epithelium, and almost all other tissues. Only the highly differentiated cell families, such as nerve and muscle cells, do not have this ability to such a great degree.

"Then rapid growth and multiplication is not the exclusive province of just cancer cells. Almost all cell families have the ability to proliferate when necessary."

"That's right, Carter."

The cell families which can't multiply rapidly are almost immune to cancer growth. However, mutant cells can occur in all tissues of your body. Mutations result from a change within certain cells that allows them to bypass their programming. These cells no longer obey their normal growth limits. They ignore the feedback controls which normally put a stop to cellular growth and reproduction after a predetermined number of cells have developed.

"Wait! I notice you haven't said anything about a virus, bacteria, germ, or any other foreign invader."

"Why should I? We're not talking about a disease here, Carter. We're talking about cancer."

"Give me a break! Our doctors and scientists are working overtime looking for the virus that causes cancer."

"They won't find it."

"Why?"

"*Cancer isn't a disease, Carter.* What you call *cancer* is simply a group of cells who are disobedient."

"I didn't realize you cells had a choice. Do you mean to tell me that cells have the ability to be obedient or disobedient?" I couldn't help being skeptical. "Are you sure you're right?" I asked suspiciously.

"Certainly, I'm right. Cancer is merely a group of disobedient cells. I said what I meant, and I meant what I said."

"All right. Don't get huffy. Explain. Disobedient to what?"

"Disobedient to the strict law of the body which says, 'Thou shalt not grow beyond they given boundaries.' This is a law that all healthy cells must obey if they want to stick around."

"I never thought of cells having 'free choice,'" I mused. "But if you cells have the ability to obey or disobey the laws, who polices you guys and keeps all the cells on the straight and narrow?"

I distinctly heard him say it. I swear to you I typed exactly what I heard. He said:

"That's my job."

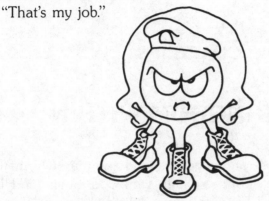

Bibliography

Antoniades, HN, and Owen, AJ: Growth Factors and Regulation of Cell Growth. Annu Rev Med, 33:445, 1982.

Bryant, PJ and Simpson, P: Intrinsic and Extrinsic Control of Growth in Developing Organs. Q Rev Biol, 59:387, 1984.

Davidson, R: Somatic Cell Genetics. New York: Van Nostrand Reinhold, 1984.

Guyton, AC: Text Book of Medical Physiology. Philadelphia: WB Saunders Co 1986.

Hall, A: Oncogenes-Implications for Human Cancer: A Review. J R Soc Med, 77:410, 1984.

Horton, JD (ed): Development and Differentation of Vertebrates. New York: Elsevier/North Holland, 1980.

Pablo, CO, and Sauer, RT: Protein-DNA Recognition. Annu Rev Biochem 53:293, 1984.

CHAPTER 3

THE KINGDOM WITHIN

"Behold, all these are kingdoms, and any man who hath seen any or the least of these hath seen God moving in His majesty and power." The words buzzed distinctly in my left ear.

"Where did you find that?" I asked. "It's beautiful!"

"It's something you read, Carter. It seems to fit, because today I'm going to introduce you to my kingdom."

"Do you mean my body?"

"Yes, but more specifically, your lymphatic system."

"I studied human physiology in college," I said. "But the only thing that really stuck with me about the lymphatic system is that whenever I get sick, the lymph nodes under my arms or in my groin swell up and hurt. I still remember the lecture my professor of physiology at the University of Utah gave on the lymphatic system. He didn't seem to know much about it though. He said something like this:

The lymphatic system has our scientists baffled. As far as our evolutionary development is concerned, we really aren't sure whether it's still evolving, or gradually disappearing. Some scientists speculate that hundreds of thousands of years ago, we had two circulation systems. Because one of the circulation systems developed a heart pump, it became more efficient than the other, thereby rendering our alternate circulation system obsolete. Some say that in another hundred thousand years, the inefficient lymphatic system will disappear completely.

Others theorize that because we're doing so well with our cardiovascular system, evolution dictates that we develop a second circulatory system. They think that perhaps a hundred thousand years from now, we'll have two cardiovascular systems servicing the body.

What I've come to think of as 'the voice' interrupted my dissertation. "Tell me, Carter, do all of your scientists teach evolution?"

"No, not all of them. But most of our scientists do support the theory of evolution."

"I don't think I'd trust a scientist who admits that he's a 'monkey's uncle.' It seems to me that as long as your men of science and medicine continue thinking of man as an 'accident,' they won't respect the inherent capability of the cells of your body to heal it without foreign substances being introduced into my environment."

"Are you talking about medicines?" I asked with a tolerant smile.

"Among other things," he answered. "Do you really think you get a headache because your body isn't producing enough aspirin?"

"There's nothing wrong with aspirin," I argued. "It's one of our most common pain-relievers. Aspirin is perfectly safe."

"Oh, really?" he retorted sarcastically. "I guess you don't know that a study conducted by doctors at Cleveland's University Hospital in Ohio has shown that aspirin compromises the infection-fighting ability of white blood cells."

"Now hold on just a darn minute," I said quickly. "Aspirin, chemically designated as acetylsalicylic acid, is a most remarkable drug from the standpoint of its physiological effects. It's our best-known and most widely-used non-biological weapon. People buy it along with their groceries. In the U.S. alone, we consume more than thirty tons of aspirin per day. To damn *aspirin* is almost like damning motherhood, you little twerp."

"Well, Carter, in spite of its palliative effects, aspirin has to be classed as essentially a 'bad' weapon when it's used consistently to cover up some trouble inside the body which really needs more fundamental attention."

"You must be wrong. Aspirin is used extensively and continuously in the treatment of arthritis," I explained.

"Oh? Do your doctors believe that arthritis occurs because the body isn't producing enough aspirin? That's obviously ridiculous, Carter. The body doesn't produce aspirin because it doesn't need aspirin. Aspirin didn't exist on this planet until 1852 when it was first made in the laboratory of a German chemist named Gerhardt."

"Look, aspirin is a very effective pain-killer. People suffering from arthritis really need it."

"But even your scientists admit that it's not clear if aspirin is either a remedy or a preventive. Aspirin doesn't effect a cure, Carter; it disguises symptoms. That interferes with my job of finding real cures."

"Yes, well. We do know that aspirin produces side effects. Indigestion, ulcers, and blood-thinning effects have been medically identified in many taking aspirin," I admitted. "But how does aspirin compromise the fighting ability of white blood cells?"

"One of the responsibilities of white blood cells is to eliminate foreign particles," he explained. "Aspirin is a foreign particle as far as we're concerned."

"I can think of hundreds of other commonly-used chemicals that are far less effective and less safe than aspirin," I countered.

"Yes, Carter, I'm only too sure that you can. And they're usually applied at the wrong time."

"What do you mean 'the wrong time?' "

"A lot of times, your doctors prescribe chemicals well after the battle has been won by the immune system. Sometimes symptoms you identify as a 'cold,' such as a sore throat, runny nose, headache, body aches, and fever, are actually the immune system at work cleaning out the dead carcasses and metabolic trash of a hard-fought internal war. The tonsils in your throat and the adenoids in your nose are drainage areas of the lymphatic system. . ."

I interrupted, "So we have post-nasal drip and mucus and our throat is scratchy."

"Right. And many times that sore throat and those inflamed tonsils and swollen lymph nodes are simply singals that the immune system is working hard at the job it was designed to do."

"I don't have my tonsils," I said.

"I know. You were four years old when your tonsils were removed. That same procedure was performed on millions of other children. Back then, most medical doctors didn't know why tonsils existed. They thought the tonsils were a leftover relic of an obsolete evolutionary process and weren't needed any longer. A lot of people don't have their tonsils, Carter. But what's really frightening is that the scientists still have the same disregard for other important parts of the lymphatic system, including lymph nodes and veins, the appendix, and adenoids."

"From your passionate defense of the lymphatic system, I'm guessing that you are more than a lymphocyte."

"I am a *T* Lymphocyte. There's a difference," he said proudly.

"What should I call you? 'Mr. T?' "

"You don't have to 'call' me, Carter. I am 'called' wherever I'm needed by 'helper' lymphocytes."

"Don't you have a name?"

"That's a human affectation. I don't need a name."

"You do, if you are going to be listed as co-author of this book."

"Oh. Okay. What do you think my name should be?"

"Gotcha! I thought you always know what I'm thinking."

"Right. 'Larry' is fine with me, Carter. Whatever makes you happy."

"Okay, Larry. Tell me what your responsibilities are."

"They are many and varied."

"Can you describe them?"

"I can do better than that, Carter. I'll take you on a tour."

"You can do that?"

"Can you type with your eyes closed?"

"Sure. With my word processor, I can correct my typos later."

"Close them."

"They are closed."

"I know."

Bibliography

Atkins, MD, RZ Dr. Atkins' Nutrition Breakthrough. New York: William Morrow and Co, Inc 1981.

Gadebusch, HJ (ed): Phagocytosis and Cellular Immunity. West Palm Beach, FL: CRC Press, 1979.

Quastel, MR (ed): Cell Biology and Immunology of Leukocyte Function. New York: Academic Press, 1979.

CHAPTER 4

THE GUIDED TOUR

As he showed me around his domain, Larry Lymphocyte let it slip that he was proud of the fact that he was part of a relatively clean body. I could see that there was plenty for him to do without having to worry about being overworked or hampered by excessive garbage blocking the areas between the cells. Everything was calm now. According to my guide, the emergency that had produced the recent flurry of excitement wasn't worth the trouble it took to get there.

Larry explained, "As a T lymphocyte, I'm ready twenty-four hours a day to protect your body every which way I can, even when the chemotoxic emergency signal sent out by the 'helper' cells over at the Command Post is only triggered by an old cell in a comfortable neighborhood passing away. Very often, by the time I arrive on the scene, a macrophage who was nearby when the aged cell died has already cleaned up the bits of nucleoprotein, organelles, and leftover cell membrane. The macrophages are the tanks of the immune system, Carter. We call that big fellow over there 'Jaws.' He really knows his job."

In spite of his awe, it was easy to see that Larry admired and liked the huge macrophage. Before I could tease him about

The Lymphatic System

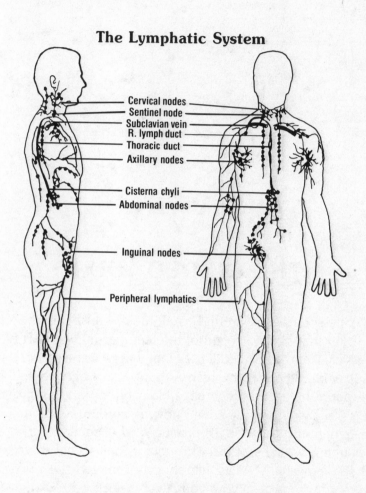

- Cervical nodes
- Sentinel node
- Subclavian vein
- R. lymph duct
- Thoracic duct
- Axillary nodes
- Cisterna chyli
- Abdominal nodes
- Inguinal nodes
- Peripheral lymphatics

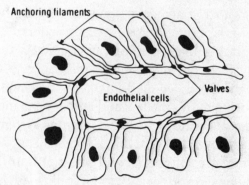

- Anchoring filaments
- Endothelial cells
- Valves

it, he was back on his soapbox.

"That's the lymphatic terminal over there, Carter, just on the other side of those tissue cells. I think I'll check out these few cells and then we'll take a tour of the node."

I followed as Larry pushed his way through the tightly-packed cells. I was surprised to feel the high level of activity that was going on inside each of these industrious chambers. Larry squeezed by some of the connective tissue which held the cells in place. Noticing a few morsels of microbes checking out a pore in one of the cells, he swooped in on them before they knew what was happening. I guess they were one of his favorite snacks. I heard him murmur, "Mmmm, good." Larry slid around another group of cells. Ever vigilant, he paused to pick up the metabolic debris that one of them had discarded.

"Everything is fine here," he remarked, looking around with satisfaction.

Suddenly, the pace picked up as we felt the suction of the terminal. With me in tow, Larry surged past the endothelial cells into the inside of the lymphatic terminal. The trap door closed behind us. As we whooshed in, I noticed that the terminal was similar to a vacuum cleaner nozzle made of overlapping cells. The cells were loosely connected in order to allow fluid and larger particles to be sucked into the lymphatic system.

Larry explained, "The lymphatic system collects lymphocytes, antibodies, certain protein molecules, and any other particles floating around the cells of the tissues that the body doesn't need. There's no turning back once you get this far, Carter. Once you enter the terminal, you're committed. From here on, it's a one-way street all the way to the node. Hang on!"

I confess to getting dizzy, but I could see that the ride really didn't bother Larry. He was obviously used to it, an old hand who had made the trip many times. Larry let me know that there's always plenty to eat inside a lymph vein, provided he could get to the tastiest bits before other lymphocytes found them. I noticed pieces of cell wall, the organelles of dead cells, and what Larry seemed to think were some delicious morsels thrown out by other cells. I even saw a bacterium or feisty virus, but I couldn't categorize it. It seemed to me that just about everything but the kitchen sink was here in the lymph vein rushing headlong toward the lymph nodes.

"Go with the flow, Carter," Larry hollered. We joined the flow of lymph fluid, sliding through small veins and one-way valves where the walls were only a single-cell thick until we emerged into larger, more spacious corridors as the veins converged. Larry indicated that he recognized some of the other lymphocytes as we rushed along, but they were too busy devouring bits of debris to acknowledge his presence.

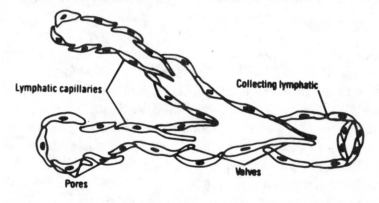

"I've worked with some of these lymphos on jobs in other parts of the body," he mentioned. "Look, there's good ol' Lorren, the one I told you we call 'Jaws,' remember? He's a beneficent beast, that old macrophage, and just about the best. He can ingest and digest over one hundred bacterium in seconds, and keep right on going. Macrophages are five times bigger and five times more deadly than the little neutrophils, another type of white blood cell.

"The last time I had the opportunity of working with Lorren was really exciting, Carter, let me tell you! There were just the three of us on site to start with, but many others were on the way. Even before the rest of them arrived, Lorren, Leonard, and I had busted through the perimeter of the cancer colony. Ol' Lorren went right into the heart of the thing and began to phagocytize those ugly mutant cells right and left! Leonard and I rubbed up against as many of the cancer cells as we could get to and injected them with deadly toxins. Those traitors literally exploded! By the time the rest of the lymphocytes converged, all that was left for them was to take over the clean-up detail.

"It's no wonder that we all admire Lorren," he continued. That magnificent macrophage is so active that you couldn't possibly guess that he's over three hundred days old. When he's gone, the force will lose a good warrior. Fortunately, ol' Jaws isn't the only good fighter we've got. The whole immune defense system is a sharp, active, aggressive fighting machine. We're dedicated to searching out and destroying any enemy of any sort that threatens our body."

I was learning a lot. Before we had gotten caught up in the pull of the terminal, Larry had done a little reminiscing for my benefit. He confided that he hadn't known what a tremendous responsibility was to be thrust upon him when he was first manufactured in the bone marrow. Along with millions of other young lymphocytes, Larry had been called to the thymus, the great school of body defense. The way he described the honor, I believe attending Thymus School must be akin to one of us being called to be an astronaut. After graduating with honors, Larry received his "T" degree. He was then assigned to an important lymph node.

The way Larry explained his weaponry showed his pride. Macrophages and neutrophils have the ability to eat the enemy. Although both are vital soldiers of the defense forces, that's their only option. But, as a T lymphocyte, Larry was given the option of poisoning invaders and enemies with hydrogen peroxide, or other toxins just as deadly, but he was also able to gobble them up like a lethal pac man.

Larry explained to me that it was his job to patrol the body and protect its identity. I couldn't help thinking that was a big job for such a small cell. But, then, he wasn't alone. The entire army of lymphocytes weighs only about two pounds, but there are about a trillion of them.

He was proud of his assigned job, but Larry modestly admitted that the lymphos couldn't take all the credit. There are many other soldiers in the defense forces of the immune system. For instance, he told me that the lymphocytes couldn't do their work without the assistance of the antibodies. He let me know that he didn't envy them their heavy responsibility either. Antibodies are the small molecules that scurry around checking the identification of each and every cell in the entire body. And, even though they are considerably smaller than the lymphos, he explained that they outnumber the lymphocytes by a million to one.

"Your forces are very well organized, Larry," I told him. "I confess, I'm really impressed."

"You ain't seen nothin' yet, Carter. There's much more for you to learn about our capabilities," he countered.

"The white blood cells and protein molecules of our vast army reach all of the tissues by using that big freeway, the bloodstream. We enter the tissues by penetrating the walls of the capillaries. Even though the pores of the capillaries are sometimes only one-tenth our size, we manage to squeeze through.

"Once we leave the bloodstream, we lymphocytes and the neutrophils are on our own. We patrol and search out intruders. We get back to our beat through the lymphatic system, our own vascular network."

"What about monocytes, Larry? Where do they fit in?"

"Monocytes are immature white blood cells circulating in the bloodstream. Monocytes are not effective as fighters, but once they leave the bloodstream, they begin to grow dramatically until they have puffed up to about five times their original size. After they are fully matured, those baby monocytes have transformed themselves into the dreaded macrophages. The macrophages usually set up camp inside the tissues spaces to protect the tissues from anything destructive to the body.

"It takes all of us working together, Carter. Teamwork, that's how it's done. For example, the antibodies move frantically from one molecule to another as they check all identification badges. Each molecule inside you humans carries an identification message known as a *epitope,* which consists of about ten letters made up of amino acids. These 'badges' stick out from each molecule and are challenged by any antigen that comes near them. If the epitope identifies the molecule as part of your body, the antibody continues on its way. If the molecule is a foreigner that the antibody recognizes, it immediately attaches itself to the invader and sends a signal to its antibody buddies to converge and attack. We T lymphocytes and the neutrophils are also tuned in to the same frequency. We proceed as fast as possible from all directions to the site of the antibody arrest.

"There's no judge or jury in here either. The fact that the molecule carries the wrong information on its epitope is proof enough for us. We white blood cells carry out immediate destruction by ingestion. The neutrophils surround, ingest, and digest the intruder without mercy. And we sensitized T cells have the ability to put another hundred lymphocytes in the area on alert. In turn, each of the hundred lymphos who answer the call also have the ability to recruit hundreds more.

"But, if it were not for the antibodies rushing around checking security badge epitopes, the lymphocyte army would find it impossible to locate all the intruders, let alone the traitors."

I stopped his dissertation to ask, "What do you mean by 'traitors,' Larry?"

"Oh, there's a rotten bunch for you," he answered scathingly. "We call those mutant cells who would be cancer 'traitors.'

They're just no good. They come from a good cell family in a good neighborhood most of the time, but good cells can go bad. Just when you least expect it, they quit obeying the Laws of Cell Division. They act like normal cells, but then they start dividing and multiplying erratically. Before you know it, there's a whole mess of 'em growing and multiplying - your doctors call it proliferating - just as fast as they can.

"If your· lymphatic system is strong, healthy, circulating properly, and kept well-informed by the antibodies, we lymphos can get in there and clean them up in no time flat. But, if the crack armies of your immune defense forces are weakened by lack of proper exercise, imperfect nutrition, or the presence of too much toxic waste in the body, the balance of power can swing in favor of the mutant cells. Then the mutants develop a law unto themselves and build a cancer colony. Give a cancer colony a few moments unnoticed in which to do its dirty work, and it will try to destroy the entire body. I shudder to think. of it!"

By the time Larry was finished with his lecture, we were fast approaching the node. I watched him check his epitope badge to make sure it was accurate. Although he had been through the lymph nodes countless times, the trip appeared to make him a little apprehensive. He indicated to me that he had learned to appreciate his security badge more and more every time he entered a node. I could feel the frenetic continuous activity of the node just ahead. We edged closer and entered through the one-way valves.

I could almost feel sorry for the bits of bacteria and viruses which had escaped the patrolling immune system forces to get this far. They had no idea of the final destruction awaiting them inside the node. The last valve opened into the hungry jaws of the millions of huge macrophages which lined the walls of the lymph node. These beneficent beasts of the immune system were hungrily waiting for their dinner, distinctly marked by the thousands of antibodies hanging all over them. I was grateful for the protection of Larry's security epitope. It would be all over for us if one of those huge macrophages grabbed us by mistake.

As he showed me around, Larry remarked with quiet pride that the node is always active. He explained that the lymph nodes of the body combined intelligence-gathering, soldier-manufacturing, and enemy-annihilation in one well-organized and very busy outpost. In a node, after being identified and stripped of its personal blueprint, scientifically known as the *antigen,* which programs it to function as an evil virus, every virus is destroyed by the macrophages. Using the virus' own antigen blueprint, the commanders of the lymph nodes direct the manufacture of an army of antibodies which will be on call to combat and destroy that specific virus if it should dare to invade the body in the future.

Because these well-trained soldiers are ever-vigilant, the body becomes immune to that particular invader forevermore. But, from the time a virus is captured and decoded, it may take as long as five days to build an army of antibodies and sensitized T lymphocytes to sufficient numbers to combat a strong invading force. This unavoidable delay in protective strength poses a danger to the body. If the virus is a particularly virulent and active strain, it could take over the entire body in less than five days. Larry explained that polio, measles, and mumps are examples of viruses which can damage the body in a short period of time.

Larry and I slipped through the node without any problems. I realized that many particles of matter were not so lucky. It seemed that all around us matter was being broken down into basic amino acids.

As we departed the node and slipped toward the huge thoracic duct in the middle of the chest, many veins poured greater quantities of lymph fluid into the larger chambers of the lymphatic system. We moved leisurely along the lymph veins, floating almost lazily in the flow of fluid being pumped by valves from one chamber to the next. Our passage reminded me somewhat of the manner in which a large ship is raised to a higher level by the means of locks.

It startled me to find that the lymph fluid was becoming milky in color, but my very able guide showed no surprise. I guess this phenomena is something that every lymphocyte gets used to. Larry explained that we were near the junction of the lymphatic system that services the small intestine. Here, the lymph fluid carries digested fat particles, along with the vitamins A and D, into the vast lymphatic network. Because fat globules and vitamin A and D molecules are too large to squeeze through the capillary membrane and enter the portal bloodstream, the only passageway of sufficient size to accommodate them is up through the thoracic duct and through the subclavian vein. Floating along through the lymphatic system, these important nutrients are delivered to the bloodstream in lymph fluid.

I could feel the surge of the thoracic duct as the final valves guarding the gates opened and closed rhythmically in concert with the action of the lungs. As the muscles of the chest worked the lungs automatically, alternately filling them with oxygen and expelling carbon dioxide into the atmosphere, large volumes of lymph fluid spurted into the fast-moving bloodstream. We were rushed forcefully into the subclavian vein.

The rest was over. I could feel Larry's excitement as he geared up to go back to work again. We slipped together into the heavy traffic of the red blood cells. Larry forgot about me for a moment as he spied a dead red blood cell right in front of him. I could tell he was hungry again. He made a beeline for the tasty morsel as other lymphocytes converged on the free meal.

I suddenly opened my eyes and watched in amazement as my fingers typed these words.

Bibliography

Fudenberg, HH and Smith, CL (eds): The Lymphocyte in Health and Disease. New York: Grune and Stratton, 1979.

Getenby, PA, et al: T-Cells, T-Cell Subsets and Immune Regulation. Aust N Z J Med, 14:89, 1984.

Guyton, AC: Text Book of Medical Physiology. Philadelphia: WB Saunders Co, 1986.

Kendall, MD: Have We Underestimated the Importance of the Thymus in Man? Experientia, 40:1181, 1984.

Sercarz, EE and Cunningham, AJ (eds): Strategies of Immune Regulation. New York: Academic Press, 1979.

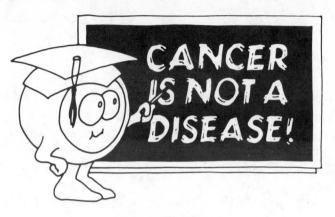

CHAPTER 5

THE DEFENSE FORCES
OF THE IMMUNE SYSTEM

"Thanks for the tour, pal-of-mine. That was quite an experience, Larry. . . and quite a story. I guess I have to agree with you that the intrigues of the CIA and the heroic deeds of the great battles of World War II pale beside the gallantry of the minute fighting forces within us."

"You might say that, Carter."

"I just did."

"So you did. And your comparison is right on target. Just as the armed forces of your nation are composed of the army, navy, marines, paratroopers, reserves, and on and on, so too are the fighting forces of the immune system made up of various divisions. For instance, our numbers consist of monocytes, neutrophils, macrophages, T lymphocytes, helper-lymphocytes, and antibodies. And there are others of us good guys who wear white hats, the white blood cells I haven't yet mentioned directly, such as the B lymphocytes. These fellows didn't go to Thymus School for their higher learning, as I did. They did their 'boning' up in Bone School to learn how to produce antibodies."

"I assume that's why they're called B lymphocytes," I inserted.

"When you're right, you're right, Carter. You have a formidable grasp of the obvious." he commented tartly.

I was a little hurt. "There's no need to get sarcastic, Larry. Are each of the cells of my internal fighting forces related to each other?"

"Well, we're sort of like cousins, I guess. But we lymphocytes can disguise ourselves and go undercover, as it were. We're the Green Berets, the fighting commandos of your immune defense forces. We can change into various other types of fighting cells, from an entire army of antibodies to huge macrophages."

I was beginning to understand. "All of the cells have to depend on each other to do their assigned tasks. What appears to be a highly sophisticated network of aggressive destruction is there for the purpose of keeping my body healthy."

"Certainly. And if your body is healthy, then my kingdom is a great place to live."

"I never thought of it quite that way."

"I know."

"Larry?"

"Yes?"

"According to your 'autobiography,' you guys destroy cancer as if there's nothing to it."

"Oh, I wouldn't say 'there's nothing to it.' We do call out the civil defense every time we come close to a cancer scare."

"Wait a minute. Are you telling me that you've had to deal with cancer yourself?"

"Yes. Several times. but nothing we couldn't handle."

"Do I have cancer now?"

"No. But there are certain signs which indicate you *could*, if you don't make some changes."

"Gee, Larry, the whole subject of cancer has to be very confusing, even to you, because there are so many different types of cancer. How are you able to keep track of all the various kinds of diseases?"

"Carter, who in your world says cancer is a disease?"

"All the doctors, scientists, the American Cancer Society. They all call cancer a disease. In fact, right here in this book written by 49 of the nation's top medical experts entitled, *The American Cancer Society Cancer Book,* it says: 'Although most of us think of cancer as a single disease, it is actually a family of more than one hundred different types all characterized by uncontrolled growth and spread of abnormal cells.' "

"Cancer is not a disease, Carter. It's a symptom."

"What do you mean, 'symptom?' A symptom is merely an outward sign of some internal malfunction."

"Exactly."

"The book says that 'cancer may be the biggest challenge faced by the medical scientist.' "

"They got that right. And as long as they have cancer misclassified, it will continue to remain both their biggest challenge *and* a major scientific mystery. Your scientists, medical doctors, authors, mass media reporters, even cancer patients, think of cancer as a whole group of diseases, because they have cancer in the wrong category. They try to treat it the same way they have very succesfully treated diseases. But, just for a moment, let us suppose that cancer is *not* a whole group of diseases. What if cancer, all types of cancer, is a symptom of a naturally occurring *condition*? How would they treat it then?"

"Hold on, Larry. This is the first time I've tried to think of cancer as nothing more than a condition. You're giving me a hard time here. What's the difference between a disease and a condition."

"Maybe I can help clarify things," Larry offered. "For the sake of this discussion, let's define 'disease' as your cells' reaction to some live thing which is 'foreign' to the body which attacks it. The sole objective of this 'foreign' invader is to live. In order to live, the invader must consume nutrients in and around the cells, or eat the cells themselves. Or, in the case of viruses, they use your cells to procreate their own kind."

"Then an example of a foreign invader attacking the body might be the bubonic plague where the disease was carried to humans by rats, and which then spread from human to human," I said, trying to sound intelligent.

"We don't have to go back to the 'Black Death' to find examples of diseases, Carter," he chided gently. "Many childhood diseases which were common to your generation are now virtually unknown, including polio, measles, mumps, smallpox, chicken pox, and even the flu."

"And diseases are contagious, right?" I asked.

"Yes, and most have an incubation period," he went on. "Pay attention now, Carter. This next point is extremely important. Any disease can be eliminated after the foreign invader is identified and destroyed."

"So what you're saying is that diseases are caused by something foreign to the body, such as germs, bacteria, viruses, and fungi. And once the scientists identify the invader, they can kill it."

"That's true. But please remember that the forces of your immune system are already attacking an invader even before you humans realize you don't feel well. And not all flora and fauna are enemies either. Your digestive system requires the help of friendly bacteria and yeasts to break down nutrients so we cells can use them."

"Larry, you and your little buddies are great. I realize I couldn't get along without you. But aren't you being a little rough on the doctors? After all, many of the diseases of the civilized world were conquered within the last two decades by our medical scientists and physicians."

"You're right, Carter. In point of fact, they did such a glorious job of wiping out so many diseases that they are attempting to use the same plan of attack against cancer. Unfortunately, they're using outmoded weapons. When they found their obsolete ammunition was useless against certain *conditions*, your medical world decided to label such conditions 'incurable diseases.' "

"Come on, Larry. Are you trying to tell me that high blood pressure, arthritis, osteoporosis, alcoholism, diabetes, and even cancer are *mislabeled* as diseases, when they really should be labeled *conditions* ?"

"Or symptoms of conditions. The next time you see a commercial on television about medication for hypertension, notice that the announcer always labels high blood pressure 'incurable.' The commercial message says the victim should 'stay on your medication because your family loves you.' "

"Of course. What's wrong with that message? High blood pressure causes strokes."

"Wrong. We cells control the blood pressure inside your body. When any group of cells in your body, such as the cells of your extremities who call your fingertips and toes home, sends out an SOS saying they are not receiving the oxygen and nutrients they need to stay alive, the heart and arteries immediately increase blood pressure to rush in emergency supplies. High blood pressure is a symptom of clogged arteries and veins, or stress."

"What causes a person to suffer a stroke, then?"

"A stroke occurs when the veins are too weak to bear the increased pressure required to get the blood to all parts of the body. I agree that high blood pressure is a dangerous condition, Carter. But it is not a disease. There is no foreign invader."

"All right, Larry. How would you suggest we handle this condition?"

"We'll talk about that later on in this book."

"What about arthritis?"

"That will be the subject of our next book."

"You are ambitious! You take on the American Cancer

Society and the AMA in this book, and still have the intestinal fortitude to announce to the world that you're taking aim at the American Arthritis Foundation next."

"I couldn't possibly have what you humans call 'intestinal fortitude,' Carter. I don't have 'guts.' I have a nucleus. But what's wrong with taking on the American Arthritis Foundation? The best your medical authorities have to offer arthritic patients is symptomatic relief in the form of a 'reduction of pain and swelling.' They still call arthritis an incurable 'disease.' "

"I suppose you have something better to offer."

"Of course. It's my job to keep your body healthy, or had you forgotten? Most arthritis is both preventable and a curable *condition,* when it's understood. But, along with the rest of the humans, you'll have to wait for the next book."

"What about osteoporosis?" I was almost afraid to challenge him, but continued, "The medical establishment says osteoporosis is an incurable disease that mainly attacks women past menopause."

"Yes, that's what they say. But are you aware that your astronauts 'caught' osteoporosis while they were up in space? They developed this so-called 'disease' because of a lack of gravity. The astronauts 'caught' osteoporosis as a result of spending time in a dramatically changed gravity-free environment outside earth's atmosphere. The cells of the bones got the message quickly. Obviously, without weight to bear, bones don't have to be as strong in space as they are here on earth. Because the bone cells weren't aware that the change was temporary, they responded to their new environment by reducing the amount of their mineral deposits.

"But, within sixty days of returning home, their osteoporosis had disappeared. The bone cells had reversed the procedure and strengthened the bones in response to the pull of gravity.

"At the risk of belaboring my point, Carter, I have to emphasize that there was no sign of a foreign invader from either outer space or inner space involved. Ergo, osteoporosis is *not* a disease and is *not* incurable, in spite of what your doctors say. Am I making myself quite clear?"

"Crystal clear, Larry. I suppose you're going to tell me next that there are other conditions which our scientists have misclassified as diseases?"

"Plenty of 'em, Carter. You'll find quite a lot of them categorized as 'old age diseases.' But our purpose in this book is to establish in your mind once and for all that cancer is *not* a disease; it's a symptom of a condition. Let me put it this way. Would you call pregnancy a 'disease?' "

"Of course not. What do you mean?"

"There are a lot of similarities between cancer and pregnancy, Carter. The cells which comprise the fetus are fast growing and proliferate rapidly. They draw a tremendous amount of nutrients from the host body, the mother, and cause many changes in homeostasis, the chemical balance of the body. Cancer does the same. But pregnancy is a controlled proliferation of cells obedient to nature's plan. Your doctors can pinpoint when conception occurred and when it will end in birth. A cancer colony, although usually slower growing than a fetus, does not follow nature's plan, the cells are disobedient and don't respond to the feedback controls, or laws, of the body. Cancer cells continue to grow at their own speed indefinitely. . . unless we can clean them up, that is."

"Wow! You've certainly presented a pretty good argument."

"Pretty good? It was great!"

"But whether cancer is called a disease or condition isn't really important, Larry. No matter how it's labeled, it's still just as deadly. As many as 462,000 Americans died of cancer in 1985," I pointed out.

"Multiply that figure by 75 trillion for the number of cells that died also."

"So what you're saying is that we're in this fight together?"

"You got that right. You die. I die."

"And you have an answer?"

"You might say that."

"Well, what is it?" I asked impatiently.

"We have to start by reeducating every one to the fact that cancer is not a disease, that it is actually a symptom of a very controllable, naturally-occurring condition."

"What difference will that make?"

"For one thing, your scientists can stop spending time and money looking for a vaccine to kill a nonexistent virus or germ. They'll be able to concentrate their efforts on ways to prevent the condition from arising, and how to identify it quickly when it does. Once your doctors accept the incontrovertible fact that cancer is a condition, their methods of treating cancer will have to change dramatically. Radiation, chemotherapy, and most surgical procedures used against cancer will pass into the history books..."

"Wait just a minute, Larry! You're talking about a major medical overhaul which will put us on a direct collision course with the American Medical Association."

"Only until they feel comfortable with the validity of the concept that cancer is a controllable condition," he answered mildly.

"But you're asking me to take the word of a tiny cell against all the mountains of evidence the scientists of the world have amassed so far," I protested.

"The word of a cell whose responsibility it is to keep you clear of cancer," he answered firmly. "You can't argue with my qualifications, Carter."

"If what you're saying is true, Larry, how can all of our scientists be so wrong?"

"They are not all wrong. Give them credit for the progress they've made. They are slowly coming to the knowledge that I live with all the time. They will eventually come to the right conclusions."

"In the meantime, millions of people are being treated as if cancer is a disease."

"A group of diseases."

"How can you explain the fact that there are so many different types of cancer then?"

"You explain to me how cancer got its name."

"What?"

"Tell me all you know about cancer."

"Not much."

"I know. This might be a good time to find out how your scientists arrived at their conclusions."

"All that information is available to us in a good medical library."

"I only have access to your memory library, Carter. Things you have experienced or read about. If the information isn't available in your memory banks, I can't help you."

"Will you give me a couple of weeks so that I can go to the library and do some research?"

"I can keep you from dying of cancer for that long."

"Thanks," I said. This time, I meant it.

Bibliography

Fischer, WL: How to Fight Cancer and Win. Canfield, Ohio: Fischer Publishing Corporation, 1987.

Guyton, AC: Text Book of Medical Physiology. Philadelphia: WB Saunders Co, 1986.

Holleb, AI, MD, (ed): The American Cancer Society Cancer Book. Garden City, New York: Doubleday and Co, 1986.

McCally, M: Hypodynamics and Hypogravics: The Physiology of Inactivity and Weightlessness. New York: Academic Press, 1969.

Sandler, H and Winter, DL: Physiological Responses of Women to Simulated Weightlessness. Springfield, VA: National Technical Information Service, 1978.

CHAPTER 6

IT'S NO WONDER CONFUSION REIGNS

'They' Say

Mass media feeds us. It feeds us every bit of information on a subject that 'they' want us to know. Unless we have access to published scientific research or medical journals, the information we have received from the media on cancer is no different. We seem to pick up the important information that 'they' want us to know almost by osmosis sometimes. And we have been well indoctrinated with the basics. 'They' say:

"Cancer is a terrible disease. One out of every four of us will die of cancer."

"Asbestos, PCBs, charcoal-broiled meats, and tobacco are all harmful carcinogens."

When we read about cancer, we are reminded that we all know friends and relatives who died of cancer. Worse, we remember several who presently have it. And it has begun to appear that the Hollywood movie stars we have enjoyed watching for so long up there on the silver screen don't age gracefully anymore. They die of cancer or AIDS.

So we put on our running shoes, hit up our friends, fellow

workers, and relatives for sponsorships and run to raise funds for the American Cancer Society. Since our government declared 'War on Cancer' in the early 1970s, it has somehow become our civic duty to run, bowl, ride bicycles, or go door-to-door to raise money to fight the common enemy, cancer.

In ancient days, leprosy was the plague that struck fear in all hearts. Cancer is the modern day equivalent of that disfiguring condition. Today, cancer is the most dreaded of all.

'We Say'

Even with all the media play, the majority of us still believe that "cancer might strike someone else, but it will never get me. And even if it should, I'll be the one to beat the odds." The scenario might go something like this:

She suspected that she might have cancer several months before she finally got her courage up and went to her doctor. After all the medical tests in the book, she thought she was ready for the worst. But when the doctor sat her down and confirmed her worst fears, the very word "cancer" made her go numb. She panicked. Confused thoughts ran through her head:

"How long do I have to live?"

"How can I prepare my family for this?"

"He might be wrong. I'll get a second opinion."

"This can't be happening to me. Not now. I'm too young."

"It isn't the end of the world."

"I'll beat it."

Nothing stimulates an interest in living more than finding yourself knocking on death's door, hoping against hope that the knock won't be answered . . . especially this way. Death by cancer is humiliating, debilitating, painful, and sometimes agonizingly slow. After your body has been subjected to the arsenal of weapons that modern medicine uses to fight cancer, it may seem that just staying alive isn't worth the effort. Be that as it may, we willingly submit ourselves to the physcial destruction of surgery, radiation, and/or chemotherapy just to gain a few more precious days of life. No matter how you perceive life and death, being a cancer patient is no picnic.

The nutritional experts in the health food industry will tell you that you should have had your picnic before you were diagnosed as having cancer. They will also tell you that if you had purchased the food supplements they offer, you might have been able to skip the whole thing.

No matter what authority you consult, confusion reigns supreme even today over the part diet plays in keeping us well. Some oncology experts say nutrition has nothing to do with the development of cancer; still others claim that eating right is the answer to cancer. While the controversy rages, nutritional laboratories comfortably straddle the middle of the road poised and ready to sell you whatever supplement the weekly news tabloids say is the latest element able to stave off the onslaught of cancer.

I'm not suggesting that health-food advocates are merely mounting money-making commercial enterprises out to catch your hard-earned dollars. Certainly there *are* some healthy cell foods available in supplement form, which we will discuss a little later. The trick is in choosing the right ones. Indiscriminate pill popping of the "element of the week" has to be risky business.

As a little more food for thought, chew on this: First, the Attorney General has determined that cigarette smoking is hazardous to your health and causes lung cancer. Second, the tobacco industry defends its position by saying that smoking cigarettes does not directly cause lung cancer. How can that be? Who's right? Does anyone really know? Who can you trust? On the one hand, the government and the American Cancer Society preach against the use of tobacco. On the other hand, the U.S. government uses tax dollars to subsidize tobacco farmers.

Medical doctors are kept abreast of the latest information

about cancer through various medical journals. Surgery, diagnosis, medications, and even correct bedside manners, are learned through medical internships. The latest diagnostic tools and advancements in medical technology are demonstrated to physicians and hospital staff personnel by representatives of the manufacturers of the devices.

The cancer specialist thinks of himself as being in the forefront of the war on cancer. He has the heavy responsibility of diagnosing a malignancy, and of informing the unlucky victim of his diagnosis. He must offer a sympathetic ear, a shoulder to cry on, and a pat on the back - not only to the patient, but to the rest of the family as well. He cannot escape developing a complex set of interrelationships with all those who are emotionally tied to the victim. The oncologist is the top gun, the general who will coordinate the battle which will be waged inside the patient's body.

Will he begin a direct frontal attack consisting of surgery? Will he bombard with radiation, or attempt to poison the cancer with chemotherapy? Maybe he will opt for a little of both, or some of each. He also takes upon himself the grave responsibility of warning the patient against succumbing to the quick-fix cancer-quacks. That warning might go something like this:

"Now that you have been diagnosed as having cancer, you will find many people will approach you with various cancer remedies and cures. And you may be tempted to fall for a published advertisement that catches your eye. Some will offer exotic formulas of herbs or esoteric vitamins. Other so-called 'cures' will demand you travel to foreign nations. The one thing all quack-cures have in common is their big-buck price tag. The 'cures' hardest to resist will be those suggested by a beloved relative or close friend. Sure, they mean well. But, trust me. None of these alternative methods work against cancer."

The medical profession seems to feel that they must shoot down what they regard as the opposition at all costs. Perhaps the reason why they guard their monopoly on the treatment of cancer is really quite simple.

Cancer is the scientist's playground. Because cancer kills, scientists have been able to request and receive billions of dollars in grants from the federal government, non-profit health-oriented organizations, major corporations, and even private sources. Phenomenal laboratories and the latest diagnostic equipment have been purchased and paid for by donations from some of the nation's largest corporations.

Today, our medical scientists *should* know more about cancer than any other health problem, considering the number of dollars that have gone into the pot. Far more bucks have been spent on the study of cancer than on anything else. According to the National Cancer Institute, the actual number of dollars expended on cancer research in 1986 totaled $113,749,600. The estimated budget for 1987 totals $123,249,300.

Millions of rats, mice, monkeys, guinea pigs, cats, dogs, and other laboratory animals have been injected with cancerous material, or implanted with growing malignancies. Our scientists have watched cancer develop, grow, divide, multiply, and proliferate wildly. We have compared our cancer cells with the cancer cells of all other countries. Science has categorized cancer by appearance, size, location, origin, and speed of reproduction. It certainly appears that the nation's experts have studied everything there is to study as far as cancer is concerned.

Our scientists should be able to tell us everything there is to know about cancer by this time. I'm sure they know, because I know. All my knowledge came from their studies. Why don't they want to share this information with us? I can't answer that. Could it be that the answer to cancer is so simple and so uncomplicated that they fear their all-important funding would dry up?

Scientists wait for laboratory tests to show solid conclusions to back up their theories. Medical doctors wait for scientific investigators to either sink or swim with the latest theories before they venture to comment.

I guess it's true that fools rush in where angels fear to tread. I am neither a scientist nor a medical doctor. And I'm certainly not an angel. The process of elimination puts me squarely in the only remaining category.

What I am is an investigative scientific reporter, so I surely can't qualify for the title of 'quack.' The worst my detractors can say of me is "The poor boy just doesn't understand." I can handle that. Comments like that, and worse, are typical of what I had to put up with when I published *The Miracles of Rebound Exercise*. That book, my first, sold over 1.3 million copies. Sales are still strong, and not only in the U.S. either. This book has been welcomed all over the world.

The knowledge that I'm going to share with you in the following chapters is simply true, and truly simple. As the scientific truths I've ferreted out are revealed in the following pages, cancer becomes so uncomplicated that you might catch yourself saying, "Ah ha!" I had that experience myself many times when I began researching the information for this book. As a long-time student of human health, I'm no different than you are.

I want to emphasize the fact that every bit of the information in this book comes from respected, authoritative, and legitimate published sources. I haven't made anything up. I haven't put anything in. I haven't even used a phrase out of context. Although this book will give you the true answer to cancer, I'm not presenting a miraculous or astounding scientific breakthrough on the treatment of cancer here. The part that's hard to believe, at least for me, is comprehending that all of the scientific, medical, and technical information in this book has been available to us (or to those of us able to understand medical terminology) for the last ten to twenty years. *In other words, the answer to cancer has been staring medical science in the face for at least a decade.*

Look, I'm not saying that I'm smarter than the finest scientific minds in the country. But I wasn't burdened with the preconceived notion that cancer is a disease either. Let me give you an example of what I mean. Science says that it is aerodynamically impossible for the bee to fly. Science says that those thin fragile gossamer wings can't possibly lift that heavy ungainly body off the ground. But those little critters aren't aware that it's scientifically impossible for them to get airborne. Fortunately for all of us who prize the products of the beehive, and I am one, the bee flies. The bees aren't burdened by preconceived scientific notions.

Finding the answer to cancer has been a matter of putting a huge puzzle together. In other words, the puzzle pieces were all there. It's just been a matter of sorting them out and fitting them in their proper places. When the final picture came clear, it seemed to me that the only alternative was to share it with you.

As you read the following chapters, I think you'll find that the knowledge presented will seem familiar somehow. The information will ring true. I'm betting that you'll be able to say to yourself at the end of each chapter, "Now, that's logical." I must warn you, however, that many of the conclusions I've reached - including the final answer to cancer - are diametrically opposed to what we've been led to believe. Nonetheless, I hope you'll enjoy reading this book just as much as I've enjoyed researching and writing it for you.

"Wow, Carter! With a little information, you really get wound up, don't you? I wonder what you'd do if you *really* knew the whole story."

"Hi, Larry. Welcome back. I haven't heard from you for awhile. Where have you been?"

"Under your skin, of course."

"I figured that."

"I was busy with that rash on your face."

"Oh, that was nothing. Just a patch of dry skin that wouldn't go away after I got sunburned."

"It was more than a sunburn, Carter."

"Was it cancer?"

"Not yet. But it could have developed into a full-fledged cancer if I hadn't called out the civil defense. Some of your cells had mutated because of the concentrated rays of the sun. But we got 'em.

"Enough chit-chat, Carter. What did we learn at the medical library?"

"Larry, you just won't believe what I found out!"

"Try me."

Bibliography

The Congressional Quarterly. April, 1986.

Statistical Abstract: US Dept of Commerce, 1987.

US Budget in Brief: Executive Office of the President, 1987.

CHAPTER 7

CANCER: PAST & PRESENT

"Well, Larry, I was surprised to find that the definition of cancer in the United Kingdom is different from the definition we use in the United States. In *Cancer, What It Is & How It's Treated,* we read: 'Cancer is the continual, uncontrolled production of cells that are of no benefit to the body.' "

Larry's reply buzzed in my left ear. "Interesting, Carter. That definition includes warts, moles, mutant cells, and all other benign growths. According to that book, everybody has cancer. One out of every million cells are mutants."

"True. And just about everyone has a wart, a mole, or other benign growth of some kind," I went on. "On this side of the ocean, the definition of cancer is different. In one of the books I checked out of the medical library, I read: 'Cancer in man is a group of related diseases (over 250) which may develop in any part of the body. It is the uncontrolled and disorderly multiplication of abnormal cells which form a malignant tumor.' "

"Which definition do you want to accept, Carter?"

"The right one, of course."

"Which one is the right one?" Larry asked mildly.

"I don't know. I never thought much about it. Does it really make a difference?"

"Only if you're serious about finding the answer to cancer."

"Do you know?"

"Of course. It's my job to know. What else did you find out at the library?"

"Well," I continued, "cancer is an ancient disease. Cancer has victimized our ancestors throughout recorded human history. Egyptian medical tracts 3500 years old describe conditions recognizable as cancer. Direct evidence includes the distinctively scarred mummies and skeletons of centuries-old cancer victims. And typical cancerous swellings and growths have been described in the medical writings of ancient Greeks, too."

"How was cancer named?"

"Early historical writings tell us that when one of these growths was removed and cut open, it had a very distinctive appearance. The growth always had a central area with channels that spread out like arms as the rapidly dividing and multiplying cells invaded healthy tissue. The ancients thought that the growth looked rather like a crab, and the Latin word for crab is *cancer*. I guess this was a very unscientific way to name a human malady. The ancient Greeks referred to cancer as a *neoplasm,* or new growth. This is also an incorrect term for the condition, although the ancients couldn't have known that it takes anywhere from five to twenty years for a cancer tumor to develop."

"That's important to remember, Carter, both in the identification of cancer and as far as your defense forces are concerned."

"Things got even more confusing as time went on. When scientists found that the cells swimming in body fluids also exhibit uncontrolled proliferation, they decided to call that *cancer* too. Today, the term cancer is applied whenever there is an abnormal proliferation of cells, even when no swelling or growth occurs. Examples include *leukemia,* an abnormal action of the blood-forming cells, and *lymphoma,* an abnormal action of the lymphatic cells."

"Although science calls these conditions cancer, the term really doesn't fit."

I could tell where Larry was leading me. "Too right," I agreed and continued. "As the scientists and medical doctors began to study cancer, they noticed that there appeared to be unexplainable and dramatic differences between the cancer afflicting each patient. Still not knowing what cancer really was, but uneasily aware that it was becoming more and more prevalent, the medical detectives began classifying it according to its primary location, the speed of its growth, its ability to spread, its individual symptoms, and its response to various types of treatment. The investigative scientists divided malignant tumors into five main classifications, with many subdivisions in each group."

The five classifications are:

Carcinomas: Carcinomas are the most common of all cancers. They arise from the tissues which cover the surface of the body or line the internal organs and passageways of the body. This is the *epithelial* tissue. Skin, intestinal, uterine, and lung cancers are all carcinomas. Subdivisions of carcinomas include several different categories, such as basal cell, transitional cell, and glandular epithelial.

Sarcomas: Sarcomas are the tumors of the connective tissues, including the muscles, bone, cartilage, and the lymphatic system. Sarcomas are also subdivided into fibrosarcomas, liposarcomas, myosarcomas, chodrosarcomas, and osteosarcomas.

Myelomas: Myleomas develop from the plasma cells which are in bone marrow.

Lymphomas: Lymphomas are found in the lymphatic system. Hodgkin's disease is an example of a lymphoma.

Leukemia: Leukemia is a cancer of the blood-forming

tissues in the bone marrow, lymph nodes, and spleen. It is characterized by the overproduction of white blood cells.

"It's certainly easy to understand how the early scientists identified cancer as a whole group of diseases, Carter."

"What do you mean, Larry?" I asked.

"Human medical doctors and scientists apparently identify diseases according to their various symptoms. But those symptoms are actually caused by a disturbance in the structure or function of an organ or organs," he explained.

"So what you're saying is that, because of the methods science uses to establish identity, they arrived at the mistaken conclusion that cancer is a whole bunch of diseases."

"That's my guess, Carter. However, all mutant cells originate from healthy cells and mimic the characteristics of their original cells," he explained. "Some cells grow slowly, while others reproduce rapidly. Since there are more than 200 different types of healthy cells in the body, it's easy to understand how your scientists were fooled into thinking that there are more than 250 different types of cancer, especially since a mutation can occur in any tissue of the body."

"So, what is cancer then?" I challenged. "A whole group of different diseases, or just one?"

"You're sliding back into the trap, Carter. You must remember that cancer is *not* a disease, it's a symptom of a condition. But, at any rate, I can understand the confusion that existed as your doctors of twenty years ago began to experience the many faces of cancer as the number of cancer patients increased. Especially since there were only two known 'cures' for cancer back then . . . surgery, or a funeral."

"You're not funny, Larry."

"You're right, Carter. Cancer is not funny. All the more reason to have the right answers."

"Are you saying that they don't have the right answers?"

"*They* don't. *We* do."

"We do?" I asked incredulously.

"Continue, Carter. What else did you learn in the library?"

"We've all heard the phrase, 'What you don't know can't hurt you,'" I said, trying to lead him into a different direction.

"I believe that is a human phrase, but it's not true, of course."

"Right. Our ignorance has already hurt, killed, and maimed millions of people, cost billions of dollars, and destroyed millions of lives. What we don't know will continue to hurt us until we fully understand our God-given physical body and the miraculous way it defends itself."

"Hooray for our side! Carter, I do believe you're beginning to see the light," he exulted.

"I'm going to tell you a horror story, Larry, about a monster worse than Frankenstein."

"Who's he?"

"I read the book, and I've seen several Frankenstein movies. You'll find him in my memory somewhere."

"Okay. I'll look him up later. Go on with your story."

"The reason this story is so terrible is because this one is true. It seems that William Steward Halstead, M.D., (1852-1922) the founder of Johns Hopkins University (Baltimore, Maryland) and a well-respected physician who practiced medicine in the late 19th century, became world famous because of a mutilating surgical procedure he devised and performed on unfortunate women who had nowhere else to turn. Many of Dr. Halstead's patients were women who were already afflicted with extremely widespread and ugly breast cancer before they came to him. These large tumors represented hygienic problems.

"Dr. Halstead developed the radical mastectomy in which the entire breast, the underarm lymph nodes, and a lot of muscles were surgically cut away. The doctor's motives were of the highest order. He developed and performed this disfiguring operation on these desperate women not in hope of effecting a cure, which he didn't believe was possible, but under the impression that the best he could offer them was the opportunity to die in relative comfort. You see, at that time, Larry, Dr. Halstead mistakenly believed that cancer cells always spread directly from the tumor to neighboring tissue."

"Boy! He didn't know much about cancer, did he?" Larry interrupted.

"We probably shouldn't really be too hard on him. Dr. Halstead knew as much about cancer as anyone else at the turn of the century," I countered. "But, he actually believed that if a patient had a lump in her breast and also a lesion in the bone of one arm, then the whole bone had to be removed at the same time as the breast was cut away. This highly-publicized operation became known as the Halstead Radical Mastectomy, or the 'en block' resection. In this procedure, the whole breast was removed, along with the muscles underneath the breast, the lymph glands and veins that drain the breast, and the lymph nodes in the armpit as well. Needless to say, an extensive skin graft was required to cover the surgical mutilation."

"It sounds to me as if the operation was worse than the cancer. Why didn't the doctor just activate the lymphatic system?"

"The lymphatic system wasn't well understood back then. And the biology of cancer was very rudimentary. Even worse, although the biological basis for the operation was known to be outmoded, as evidenced by research conducted in the early 1940s, the very same procedure was considered the only viable surgical option available against breast cancer until the late 1970s. And it took a television show to bring the problem to the attention of the public. Halstead's Radical Mastectomy versus the Lumpectomy, where only the lump of cancerous growth itself is removed, was hotly debated on the Merv Griffin Show in 1979."

"That's a lot of cutting and slicing."

"Please, Larry. Let's not get morbid."

"Most of that surgery was totally unnecessary, Carter!" he said sternly.

"How do you know, Larry. You weren't there."

"It's my job to know, you dunderhead! Haven't you been paying attention?"

"But the operation did work, Larry," I said lamely. "There was no known cure for breast cancer before 1894. It wasn't until 1945 that the National Cancer Institute announced that it was possible to cure 45 percent of all women with breast cancer."

"I'm almost afraid to ask. What happened to the other 65 percent, Carter?"

"They died of their cancers, I guess."

"That doesn't sound like a resounding success rate to me."

"But, Larry *all* of them would have died if they hadn't had the surgery," I protested.

"How do you know, Carter. You weren't there."

"You're right. But for the first 60 years of this century, there was no way to determine if a surgical procedure as mutilating as the radical mastectomy was necessary for *all* patients. We just didn't have the concrete scientific documentation we needed to make an accurate determination. However, science now says that a simple mastectomy, the removal of breast tissue only, and sometimes even a simple lumpectomy, is just as likely to cure patients of breast cancer without the disability and cosmetic disfiguration caused by Halstead's radical procedure."

"That's what I've been talking about, Carter. Ignorance is a killer, no matter how intelligent your human scientists and medical doctors profess to be."

"Larry, it takes a long time to learn. Besides, the development of successful surgical procedures against breast, colon, and other cancers had to wait for the development of modern medical technologies, such as blood transfusions, new anesthetics, improved surgical techniques, and chemical antibiotics."

"Nothing takes the place of prevention, Carter. There is just no logical reason for a human to die of cancer."

"Now, that's quite a mouthful, Larry."

"I don't have a mouth."

"Figure of speech."

"I don't speak."

"Stop contradicting me. Did you like the story?" I asked.

"Scary."

"I'm only just beginning. Let me tell you another one that will really curl your hair."

"I don't have hair."

"I'll ignore that remark," I said sternly. "To continue, Wilhelm Conrad Roentgen (1845-1923) earned the first Nobel Prize ever awarded for Physics in 1901 for his 1895 discovery of x-rays."

" 'X' what?"

"X-rays. When Roentgen discovered that x-rays penetrate the tissues of the body like a light beam, this new discovery was quickly recognized as a superior tool for the diagnosis of broken bones and other internal problems."

"Sort of like bugging a room with surveillance equipment."

"You might say that. But, there was trouble in paradise. As time passed, science discovered that x-rays also destroyed cells."

"Oh, no!"

"In this case, that's good, Larry. When a tumor was bombarded with x-rays, the tumor shrank as its cells were blasted out of existence."

"But, Carter, that means that the healthy cells that were in the path of the x-rays were also destroyed."

"Unfortunately, yes. But some healthy cells have to be sacrificed in order to kill cancerous cells, Larry," I chided. "True x-rays come from a cathode ray tube, which is man-made. But the gamma rays given off by cobalt and cesium have the same ability."

"The ability to kill cells."

"Right," I agreed. "The x-ray machines developed in the

1920s and 1930s operated with a low voltage of around 250 kilovolts. These machines resulted in a significant burning of the skin's surface, making treatment very difficult to bear."

"Harder to hide the damage, too," Larry remarked sarcastically.

I ignored him and went plodding on. "But science was working on that problem. Supervoltage equipment came next, including the cobalt units and linear accelerators."

"Which kill cells more efficiently,"

"They deliver super-large doses of radiation to the tumor, with only minimal damage to the superficial tissue that's in the way."

"Easier to hide the damage," Larry remarked disgustedly.

"Be fair, Larry. The scientists are aware that radiation affects normal tissue, but their understanding of cancer is incomplete. The medical experts universally agree that surgery and radiation therapy are both localized forms of treatment which, unfortunately, must kill normal cells in order to kill cancer cells."

"Carter, even *minimal* damage to healthy cells is not acceptable. That's my family you're talking about and your body. Are you telling me that total destruction of all the cells in the area is okay, just as long as the tumor is destroyed in the process?"

"I guess I am."

"Pardon my sarcasm, Carter. But that's like throwing a hand grenade into a roomful of school children because a terrorist is holding them hostage inside."

"There's sound logic behind the theory, Larry. If the tumor is sensitive to the effects of the radiation, the treatment will destroy cancer cells before permanent damage can occur to normal tissue."

"What if the tumor isn't radiosensitive?" he asked.

"Well, I guess the dose of radiation required to destroy cancer cells kills normal cells as well."

"In other words, total destruction of all cells in the area is okay, just as long as the tumor is destroyed in the process?"

"So the American Cancer Institute preaches."

"I don't care for their thinking."

"They're not out to get *you*, you know. Don't take it personally, Larry."

"How can I take it any other way, Carter? I'm one of the innocent cells who's being shot at."

"I've got another story that will curl your hair."

"I don't have hair, Carter."

"Stop complaining. A lot of cancer patients don't have hair either," I said tartly. "Even I had a hard time believing this next story. It's easy for us to assume that the mice scientists use to test chemicals that might work against cancer are like the common field mouse. But nothing could be further from the truth."

"Please elaborate."

"Sure. Before 1916, cancer mouse models did not exist. It was impossible to test possible cancer drugs for efficacy before giving them to a human cancer patient. So a mouse ideal for cancer research was developed in the laboratory. This was a special strain of mice with part of their immune system removed."

"So human cancer can be grown in this strain of mice, I presume."

"You're ahead of me Larry. Because this strain of hairless mice doesn't have a normally-functioning immune system, yes, a human tumor can actually be transplanted under the skin and grown in one of the little creatures. Scientists are now able to test drugs against human tumors by growing them in nude mice."

"If the mice had their immune system intact, this would be impossible."

"Exactly."

"Let me get this straight," said Larry. "Almost all cancer research has been done on mice that have been genetically stripped of their natural immune capabilities?"

"All in the name of science," I agreed.

"That's like taking the rifles away from the army and then sending them out to fight a battle to the death."

"You have to understand, Larry. The scientists didn't want the immune system to win. That's the only way they can test other alternatives."

"I don't understand humans," he said sadly.

"I'm almost beginning to agree with you," I confided. "This is the part that gets really scary. During World War II, an accidental explosion of mustard gasses in Naples harbor killed many people. Autopsies revealed that these people died because their immune systems atrophied and some of their bone marrow cells had disappeared. The scientists thought that perhaps cancers originating in these types of tissues might be effectively treated with the chemicals in mustard gas."

"Somehow the logic of that escapes me."

"Nonetheless, back in 1950, Congress gave the National Cancer Institute five million dollars to start a cancer drug development program. This program has been responsible for most of the cancer drugs that are now in use."

"Where does the NCI get the chemicals they test for activity against human cancers?" he asked.

"Sometimes a scientist has a bright idea for a drug that might interfere with cellular growth and formulates a chemical combination from scratch. Or a known chemical that a scientist thinks might possibly have an adverse effect on cancer is chosen for testing."

"Where do all these chemicals come from?"

"There are about 200,000 new chemicals recognized worldwide every year," I explained. "Any one of these compounds might qualify as a cancer drug. Obviously, not all of these chemicals have been tested. But, since 1955 when the cancer drug development program began, 500,000 compounds have been screened. Of the 40 cancer drugs currently around, 26 of them are commercially available."

"What properties must a drug show to be accepted by the National Cancer Institute as a cancer drug?"

"Any chemical that interferes with the mechanism of natural cell division is a candidate. Most cancer drugs interact with the genetic material in a cell."

"So, anything that keeps cells from dividing naturally might be classed as a cancer drug?"

"That appears to be the case. Let's look at some of them:"

Mustard Gas: Mustard gas (dichlorodiethyl sulfide) is a highly toxic war gas which causes conjunctivitis and blindness. Its vapor is extremely poisonous and can be absorbed through the skin. Mustard gas is also used medicinally to treat cancer. But it *causes* cancer of the bronchi in industry workers exposed to it, and causes cancer of the lungs, larynx, trachea, and bronchi in cancer patients treated with it.

Nitrogen Mustard: Chemotherapeutic alkylating agents were discovered while scientists were conducting secret research during World War II, but the full story was not revealed until 1963. It seems that the sensitivity of normal lymphoid tissue to the cytotoxic (cell killing) action of nitrogen mustards led to a test on one mouse with a transplanted lymphoma. The encouraging results of that test led to more extensive investigation. Eventually, related compounds were developed for clinical use in the treatment of malignancies, including busulfan (Myleran), cyclophosphamide (Cytoxan), Leukeran, and L-phenylalanine mustard (Melphalan).

But the nitrogen mustards cause cancer when injected or given intravenously to mice in even very small doses. Unfortunately, many of the cytotoxic drugs have been found to cause cancer years after being used to combat cancer.

5-Fluorouricil: This compound is produced by placing fluorine on a normal pyrimidine, creating a fraudulent DNA building block. In the cells of the body, this chemical interferes with an enzyme that the body requires to build DNA. Because

DNA cannot be produced, the cell cannot divide.

Methotrexate: An anti-vitamin, this drug masquerades as folic acid, an important part of B complex. Because the cell cannot function without folic acid, it dies.

Procarbazine: In technical terms, procarbazine depolymerizes DNA. In nontechnical terms, this drug nicks the DNA and breaks it. Without DNA, a cell cannot reproduce.

Bacterial Compounds: Part of the bacterial defense system includes substances that bacteria put into their surroundings to prevent other bacteria from growing. These substances slip between the strands of DNA and prevent its copying functions from working. Drugs produced from bacteria include *adrinmysin, daunomycin, dactinomycin,* and *mithramycin.*

L-Asparaginase: L-Asparaginase is an enzyme which breaks down asparagine, an amino acid which is an essential building block in proteins. Without asparagine, the cell cannot produce protein and literally starves to death.

Vincristine & Vinblastine: These chemical compounds were derived from the *vinca roseacea* plant, a common ground cover which grows happily in many areas all over the country, including my backyard. Originally, vincristine and vinblastine were developed for the treatment of diabetes. When the scientists noticed these compounds killed cells, they were reclassified as cancer drugs. These two chemicals produce mitotic arrest, thereby making it impossible for cells to divide and multiply.

"Chemotherapy, the use of drugs to kill cancer, is an undeniably expensive proposition, both in terms of dollars expended and in terms of cost to the body," I acknowledged. "Because the chemicals attack all quickly-dividing cells, healthy as well as malignant, the patient treated with chemotherapeutic drugs pays a high price indeed. The side effects of these chemicals are devastating!"

"But, Carter, all of these chemicals spell death to the lymphocytes, antibodies, and neutrophils of the immune defense forces!" exclaimed Larry in disbelief. "When we identify cancer cells inside the body, it's the white blood cells of the immune system which are the ones multiplying and dividing the fastest in order to fight the cancer."

"I agree with you, Larry, and that's only part of it. Chemotherapy, as well as radiation therapy, both kill normal cells in the bone marrow and in the digestive tract. Serious side effects, such as diarrhea, vomiting, anemia, and a loss of hair, result. But it can't be helped, I guess."

"Oh, yes it can," he protested vehemently. "These side effects are merely inconveniences and cause minor discomfort to you humans, but they mean death to me and millions of my buddies as well."

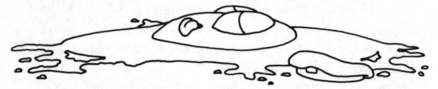

"These treatments can also mean death to the patient."

"Of course, Carter. Clearly, destroying too many normal cells can cause the patient to virtually self-destruct. But the killing of healthy cells is not necessary when you really understand cancer."

"I suppose that's true. In fact, the degree to which chemotherapy actually increases cure rates or extends useful life for cancer patients is still debated by the cancer experts themselves."

"There's still another problem to be considered, Carter. Cancer cells are notorious for changing their characteristics. Those ugly traitors can become resistant to even the most powerful of your chemicals. Such resistance is the result of the mutations that occur, on average, only once among many millions of cancer cells. But once is enough. Because cancerous tumors contain billions of cells, there is always the possibility that one cell will sustain the mutation that makes it and its descendants forever resistant to a particular drug."

"I never thought of that," I admitted.

"There's more," Larry cautioned. "Because all chemotherapeutic drugs are mutagens themselves, they may actually increase the rate at which resistant mutants appear. The drug may actually favor the mutations by destroying the cells which are sensitive to the drug. Eventually, the resistant mutants will multiply and form a drug-resistant cancer that no chemical can touch. And with the immune system out of commission . . ."

"That will make things even worse."

"Cool down, Larry. The doctors are just trying to help."

"Are you sure? It doesn't sound to me as if they've helped very much so far. They've just confused the issue."

"That's a wild accusation, Larry," I said sternly.

"All right," he said patiently, "let's go back over the history of cancer and find out if I'm right."

"Okay. Let's see." I referred to my notes. "Where were we? Oh, yes. On December 9, 1969, a full-page ad in the *New York Times* really got the public stirred up by suggesting that a cure for cancer was at hand."

"Great!" he enthused. "That would certainly make my life easier."

"The ad was prepared by an elite group of five who called themselves the Citizens Committee for the Conquest of Cancer. They said, 'There is not a doubt in the minds of our cancer researchers that the final answer to cancer can be found.' The ad quoted a former president of the American Cancer Society as saying, 'We are so close to the cure for cancer that all that is needed to guarantee it is the will and the kind of money and comprehensive planning that went into putting a man on the moon.' With that kind of serious effort, the Committee assured us, 'a cure for cancer by 1976 is a distinct possibility.' "

"Hmmm," Larry said thoughtfully. "From 1969 to 1976 is

seven years. That should be enough time for any scientific organization to understand cancer. What happened?"

"Quite a bit. By the end of 1971, President Richard Nixon actually declared war on cancer by signing the National Cancer Act into law, and the taxpayer-financed crusade against cancer got underway."

"Well, that should have provided plenty of money for the effort."

"Yes, it did. It not only provided tax dollars, but the National Cancer Institute in Bethesda, Maryland, formed in 1938, was transformed into a giant monolithic superagency. The NCI was made responsible for directing cancer research through its burgeoning staff of bureaucrat/scientists. Since then, the NCI has spent over ten billion dollars funding cancer research. Congress now appropriates about 800 million dollars annually to help finance the war against cancer."

"How much you humans spend doesn't impress me. Carter. It's the *results* that are important. What about the results?"

"Unfortunately, Larry, the billions and billions of dollars we've poured into cancer research programs has had little or no effect in preventing or eliminating cancer. In the U.S. alone, the cancer death rate has risen from approximately 120,000 persons in 1930 to 480,000 cancer-caused deaths in 1985."

"Carter, that's terrible! Your government must have a way to control what looks like massive boondoggling, ineptness, and stagnation."

"I just wish we did. You see, Larry, when a governmental agency gets too big, it sort of runs itself."

"That sounds like a 'cancer' to me," Larry observed sternly,

"The excuse the NCI gives to the American public is that they are attempting to unravel the mysteries of the abnormal cellular behavior that leads to cancer. At best, it's an endless process, and they're just beginning."

"They're wasting time, Carter. You humans don't have to know everything that causes cancer," he answered scornfully.

Even I don't know *why* a cell mutates. All any of us have to know is how to get rid of a mutation after it happens."

"Dr. Samuel Epstein, the author of *The Politics of Cancer* just happens to agree with you, Larry. Dr. Epstein says, 'The number one priority job of the NCI has to be cancer prevention.' "

"Smart man! Now we're getting somewhere!"

"Not really. Dr. Epstein feels that the entire decision-making apparatus of the NCI is slanted in favor of chemotherapy and basic research."

"That's easy. Can't the NCI be directed to concentrate on cancer prevention?"

"Unless Congress takes charge and insists on overseeing their policies, I'm afraid the NCI will never change."

"Surely the American people can see what's gone wrong."

"I wish it were as easy as that. Instead of concrete results based on effective research and clinical practice, the NCI just continues making stale claims. By a kind of verbal slight-of-hand, their periodic announcements to the public transform 20 years of ineffectual work into an illusion of progress.

"Let me give you an example of what I mean, Larry. In June of 1977, during a congressional investigation of the cancer program, it was pointed out that Frank J. Raucher, Ph.D., the former head of the National Cancer Institute, and Dr. R.L. Clark, president of the American Cancer Society, coauthored an article which was published in *The Washington Post*. The article stated that one out of every three cancer victims was being cured as a result of solid progress in cancer research. Congressman John W. Wydler of New York, then the ranking minority member of the Subcommittee under the auspices of the House Committee on Government Operations, pointed out that in 1957, twenty years before, the same proportion of cancer cases - one in three - was being cured.

"And in 1985, eight years later, the American Cancer Society cheerily informed us that, 'Three out of every eight patients who develop cancer this year will be alive five years after diagnosis.' But this doesn't represent a lengthening of the lifespan of a cancer victim. It merely reflects technological improvements in methods of medical diagnosis."

"Wow, Carter! That doesn't sound very impressive for the NCI or the ACS people, does it?"

"I guess not, Larry. In spite of a continuing campaign mounted by the leaders of the cancer establishment in an attempt to hoodwink the public into believing that advances are being made in the so-called 'war against cancer,' objective experts tell us in a frank evaluation that the National Cancer Program is really a devastating failure. In fact, this NCI-produced fiasco has wasted billions of taxpayers' dollars on predictably worthless cancer programs. Some, like the mammography breast-screening program for women, have turned out to be high-risk health hazards.

"And millions of trusting cancer patients have been sacrificed to ineffective treatments which were often deadlier than the cancer itself. The NCI has stubbornly persisted in pursuing these expensive and dangerous therapies, in spite of the fact that these well-established truths have been published in the NCI's own publications. They know, for example, that their tragic preoccupation with relatively ineffective and exceedingly harmful chemotherapeutic cancer agents, which have been approved by the Food & Drug Administration for use or testing on human patients, are highly toxic at applied dosages. They markedly suppress the immune system, which inhibits the patient's native resistance to a variety of diseases, including cancer. They are also highly carcinogenic, meaning that these chemicals produce cancers in a wide variety of body organs.

"Larry, during my research, I visited a chemotherapy ward. It's sad to see youngsters with their gums bleeding and their hair falling out, and know that their intestines are full of bleeding lesions, making it impossible for them to evacuate their bowels. Their skin hangs in folds and flakes off in patches. Their teeth get loose, they vomit, and, because these chemicals are so toxic, they feel absolutely miserable. And, because cytotoxic drugs often cause secondary cancers to develop as well, chemotherapy isn't a cure. Its effects are far worse than the cancer itself.

"In fact, a study published in the *New England Journal of Medicine* in 1984 reached the conclusion that colon cancer victims don't live any longer when they receive chemotherapy along with the standard surgical removal of their tumors. This 70-week long trial followed the treatment of 572 patients in 13 different hospitals. It was conducted by the Gastrointestinal Tumor Study Group of the Roswell Park Memorial Institute in Buffalo, New York."

"Carter, it sounds to me as if it's not only the cancer patients who are sick, the whole system is sick. It's time for a major overhaul of the whole cancer research program."

"That's easier said than done, Larry. Ever since the latter months of 1971, which is when Congress commissioned the National Cancer Institute to lead the war on cancer, the NCI has had almost unlimited powers to parcel out vast sums of money for research. This factor has created a group of kingmakers, sort of godparents, of the NCI. The kingmakers make certain that the so-called 'right people' end up in positions of power on the country's top-drawer advisory boards, like the President's Cancer Panel.

"An article in the December 1983 issue of *Science Magazine* pinpointed the problem. In essence, it stated that too few people, all on intimate and friendly terms with each other, are in charge of handing out large sums of money each to the other."

"Carter, I've seen cancer before and I know how it works. I see cancer now."

"You might be right, Larry. It surprised me to discover that the way NCI cancer researchers are expected to choose subjects for their experiments is based on a 'play-the-winner' policy.

NCI researchers select only those who have the best chance of surviving. That way, better results can be reported in the medical journals."

"The bottom line is that both chemotherapy and radiation are so harsh that they sometimes cause a second cancer, even while destroying the first," Larry said angrily.

"The scientists are trying to eliminate that problem," I said defensively. "Some of our top cancer experts believe that our greatest hope is to devise drugs that will selectively destroy cancer cells only, without harming normal cells . . . a sort of 'magic bullet' against cancer."

"Carter, that's where I come in."

"What do you mean?"

"I already have the magic bullet."

"You do?" I exclaimed in astonishment.

"Yes. It's called hydrogen peroxide."

"Come on! You don't mean that same stuff we buy in quart bottles in the drug store to clean wounds? That's too simple."

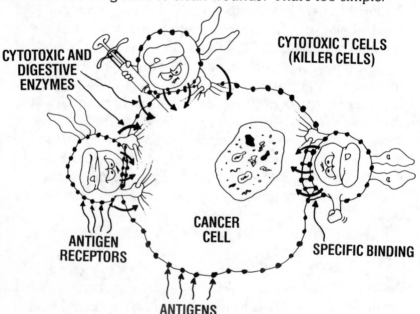

"The very same. Why do you use hydrogen peroxide to clean wounds, Carter?"

"Because it kills germs, of course."

"What are 'germs' "

"Germs are microscopic single-celled organisms..."

"Hydrogen peroxide is a perfect cell poison. We T lymphocytes manufacture it ourselves. It kills all kinds of cells, including cancer cells. And, if it doesn't work, I've got superoxide and hydroxyl ions I can use on them. All these cell poisons are lethal to most bacteria and cancer cells in even very small quantities. How do the human scientists plan to find a chemical which can qualify as a magic bullet?"

"I admit that it seems unlikely that simply screening an endless series of chemicals for anticancer activity will ever yield a powerful and highly-selective drug," I said reluctantly. "The haystack is immense, and the needle is very small, perhaps even illusory."

"I agree with you," Larry answered and proceeded to hammer home his point. "Even if they do finally find such a chemical, how do they plan to deliver it to cancer cells only?"

"There's been talk about pulling lymphocytes already sensitized to a particular cancer colony out of the body, growing them in a tissue culture, and then reintroducing them into the body in large numbers by transfusion."

"I'll bet your doctors will charge a lot of money for that process," Larry prodded.

"Of course," I agreed. "That's their job."

"No, it isn't. That's *my* job. What's more, I do it free and I do it a lot faster than they can," he said angrily. "I've had enough, Carter. You're making me sick. I can see that humans are no different than cells. It seems to me that even the best-intentioned organizations go out of control because even humans mutate under the right conditions. I'll be back to continue our discussion, but right now I need to refresh myself with a trip through the node where order reigns supreme and humans can't confuse the issues."

Bibliography

Devita, BT: Cancer Treatment. US Department of Health and Human Services.

Guyton, AC: Text Book of Medical Physiology. Philadelphia: WB Saunders Co, 1986.

Laws, PW: X-Rays - More Harm than Good? Emmaus, PA: Rodale, 1977.

Morra, M and Potts, A: Choices, Realistic Alternatives in Cancer Treatment. New York: Avon Books, 1980.

Null, G and Steinman, L: A Billion Dollar Boondoggle. New York: Penthouse, 1985.

Salsbury, KH and Johnson, EL: Indispensable Cancer Handbook. New York: Seaview Books, 1981.

Smedley, H, Sikora, K and Stepney, R: Cancer, What It Is and How It's Treated. Oxford, Great Britain: Basil Blackwell Ltd, 1985.

Washington Post, Washington DC: 1977.

Winter, R: Cancer Causing Agents. New York: Crown Publishers Inc, 1979.

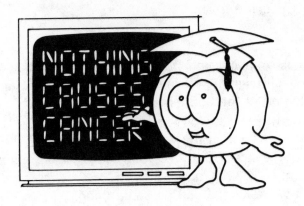

CHAPTER 8

LARRY EXPLAINS
WHAT CAUSES CANCER

"Okay, Larry. You're on. Since you're a T lymphocyte, have access to my thoughts and emotions, and are in constant communication with my immune defense forces, surely *you* must know exactly what cancer is. I've done what you asked. I've spent months in public libraries and medical libraries and university libraries exhaustively researching the subject. I don't think there's a medical book or scientific journal or research paper or magazine article or newspaper report even remotely connected to cancer that I haven't dug up and pored over. I've reported to you exactly what humans think cancer is, how it was named, and told you some of the ways that our medical and scientific authorities are combating it. I've done my part. Now, I'm asking you to make good on your promise. What is cancer?"

"Carter, I thought you'd never ask."

"Larry, I thought that was the purpose of this whole book."

"Are you sure you're ready for this?"

"After that last chapter, I think I'm ready for anything."

"I'll try to put it in terms you can understand, Carter. Here goes: Unlike malaria and polio, for example, cancer is *not* caused by a foreign organism that enters the body. Cancer is an innate part of the body. In a true sense, every human is predisposed to cancer."

"So. . . everyone in the world has cancer?"

"No, not cancer. But everyone does have mutant or disobedient cells."

"Aren't we talking about the same thing?"

"Not at all. Mutant cells and cancer are as different as an egg and a chicken."

"You mean that mutant cells might be compared to an egg."

"Yes. You might say that the egg is a 'pre-chicken' condition. In the same way, a mutant cell is considered a 'pre-cancerous' condition. It's just as normal for a human to have mutant cells as it is for a human to have a baby. Both are normal conditons of the body."

"You make it sound so simple, Larry. Understanding cancer just can't be as easy as all that."

"Why not? When your scientists finally understood everything there was to know about smallpox, it was easily controlled. The same concept can be applied to eradicating cancer," he said reasonably.

"First, a mutation occurs when something happens to certain normal genes inside your cells. The genes that have mutating potential are called *proto-oncogenes.* In your scientific terminology, that translates to pre-cancerous genes. What transforms them into *oncogenes,* or true mutant cancer genes, can be almost any foreign substance introduced into your internal environment in the air you breathe or the food you eat, or the mutation can simply be a spontaneous change with no identifiable cause."

"But you're not talking about cancer *cells.*"

"No. These are parts of the DNA inside the cells."

"Yes, of course," I answered thoughtfully. "My study of these piles of research papers here on my desk indicates that our experts have suspected that genes have something to do with the development of cancer for quite a while, Larry. But, until they developed the technology they needed to manipulate genes, they weren't able to confirm this hypothesis. Research groups led by Robert Weinberg of MIT and Michael Wigler of Cold Spring Harbor Laboratory pulled the DNA out of a human bladder cancer cell and inserted it into healthy mouse cells they had growing in test tubes. The mouse cells turned cancerous. By testing smaller and smaller segments of the cancerous DNA, they were finally able to pinpoint the gene responsible for the cancer."

"There! You see! Your human scientists are coming around. Give them time. Remember though, the genes of all the cells of the body are not necessarily oncogenes. Something has to happen before a healthy cell turns into a traitor."

"What are you talking about, Larry? Bribery?" I joked. "That's one way to turn a good person bad."

"Bribery won't do it, Carter. Your cells are not paid to keep you healthy," he answered seriously.

"I see. You mean they're good-for-nothing," I said, trying to keep a straight face. He didn't understand my human humor.

"There are three different processes that can transform a normal gene into an oncogene," he explained patiently. "The DNA, the blueprint of the cell, is built of very precise building blocks that your scientists call *nucleotides*. If one nucleotide is substituted for another in the process of cell duplication, this is called *point mutation*. When this happens, a mutant cell results.

"The second process is called *chromosomal translocation* and occurs when chromosomes of the cell swap a chunk of genetic material with each other."

"I remember from my studies that 100 percent of patients with Burkitt's Lymphoma, a cancer that chiefly affects children, exhibit a chromosomal translocation." I was rather pleased to be able to offer this bit of information I had stored away in my brain.

"That's right, Carter. But let me continue, please. The third process is called *amplification*. Cells have the ability to amplify their copying function, meaning that they make multiple copies of genes. Instead of making two copies of a certain gene per cell in preparation for division, a cell may manufacture hundreds."

"I remember reading that scientists in San Francisco have reported finding a thirty-to-fifty-fold increase in oncogenes," I inserted.

"Your memory is better than I thought, Carter."

"I just read about it last week," I acknowledged.

"Still, Carter, it's actually very hard for a mutant cell to qualify as a legitimate potential cancer cell."

"Why is that?"

"One mutation will not do it. A cell has to mutate twice. In every instance, cancer cells are caused by mutations of the genes in the DNA that control both *cell growth* and *cell reproduction*. But, even then a cancerous tumor doesn't develop unless cell proliferation goes out of control. For example, if just one oncogene is produced early in life, the threat of cancer won't surface until a second gene is disrupted and turns into an oncogene itself."

I was beginning to understand. "So that's why it may take twenty years or more before a cancer is detectable. What causes a genetic mixup to occur in the first place?"

"Anything that alters DNA has the potential to produce oncogenes. Radiation treatments, chemotherapy, and chemical carcinogens have all been shown to have that ability. Chemical substances of certain types also have a high propensity for causing mutations, including aniline dye derivatives, asbestos, and the tars, toxins, and nicotine in cigarette smoke.

"There's more," he continued. "Physical irritations, including the continuing abrasion of the lining of the intestinal tract by some foods, or even abrasions on the outside of the body, can lead to more rapid cellular production as the body tries to remedy the damage. And fast cellular production offers a greater chance for mutations to occur."

"Let me get this straight in my mind, Larry. For me to have cancer, a cell has to mutate twice, and then develop into a colony that grows unchecked. That doesn't sound very hard."

"In a healthy body, it's close to impossible."

"Oh? Why is that?"

"First of all, most cell mutations have less survival capability than normal cells and simply die. Second, only a very few of the mutated cells that manage to survive actually disobey the normal feedback controls that prevent excessive growth. They live out their limited lifespan as noninvasive mutant cells until they die of old age. And, third, those cells that are potentially cancerous are the target of search and destroy teams of, pardon my pride, your immune system. We usually manage to clean up deviant cells long before they can grow into a cancer colony."

"It must be hard for you to tell the difference between a mutant cell and a normal cell," I remarked.

"You keep forgetting that knowing the difference is an important part of my job, Carter. You see, most mutated cells form abnormal proteins within themselves because of their altered genes. As the true guardians of your body, we know exactly which proteins belong to your body, and which ones do not. The presence of an abnormal protein tells the B lymphocytes that they need to form an army of antibodies to destroy the renegade cells."

"That's great. I see that I owe you my very life," I said with real enthusiasm. "But is the tendency to develop cancer genetic then?" I asked.

"No. If a mutation should occur before conception, it will show up as a birth defect. Cancer is not generally inherited in the way that cystic fibrosis or hemophilia are. In most cases, the damage to the genes occurs after birth. However, families can exhibit a strong inherited predisposition to cancer. Remember, two mutations must take place before cancer arises. In certain families, one or more of the oncogenes can be inherited, meaning that it takes far fewer mutations for a renegade to develop," he explained.

"What else causes cancer?"

"Nothing."

"*Nothing!* That can't be right. How about viruses?"

"Viruses can produce mutant cells in both humans and animals, but the number of human cell mutations is fairly small."

"But, Larry," I objected strongly, "our scientists can control viruses in the laboratory. The way viruses exert a carcinogenic effect has taught us more about the processes that underline all forms of cancer than all the studies of physical and chemical agents combined."

"That's because a virus is a single piece of DNA, Carter, a collection of genes protected by a protein coat. A virus doesn't have the other structures normally found in cells. It doesn't have the machinery to build proteins, so it can't reproduce its own. To do this, it must invade a host cell. The virus attaches itself to the cell membrane and transfers its genes inside. Once it gets inside, the virus takes over the reproducing function of the cell. Instead of producing proteins, it starts to produce copies of the viral genetic material."

"What's this about a 'protective coat?' "

"The virus genes instruct the host cell to produce a protective coat of proteins. After a while, a complete new set of virus particles are formed. These particles emerge and move on to infect other cells."

"There!" I said triumphantly. "We have learned a lot about viruses and genes. . ."

"But nothing about what causes cancer," he countered quickly.

"Not true, Larry. Our scientists have tagged thousands of things that cause cancer. As a matter of fact, there are scads of books about all the things that cause cancer." I picked up several from the stack on my desk. "Here's one . . . here's another . . ."

He interrupted quickly. "Carter, your books are full of various chemicals and elements which your human scientists tag 'mutagenic' or 'carcinogenic.' Actually, there are no chemicals, agents, or elements which can accurately be termed cancer-causing, or carcinogenic."

"Carcinogenic or mutagenic. What's the difference?"

"Nothing."

"So how many things listed in our books really do cause cancer?"

"Not one."

"I don't understand."

"You're not alone, Carter. Nobody else understands either, including your men of science and medicine."

"Larry," I said sternly, "I believe an explanation is in order here."

"Are you ready for this?"

"*Yes!*" I hollered in exasperation. "What causes cancer?"

"Nothing *causes* cancer, Carter. But an inefficient immune system allows cancer to develop."

"Just like that?" I said in exasperation. "If you're going to continue giving dumb messages to me, don't expect me to write them down and then publish them. Humans aren't stupid, Larry. Do you really think the whole world is going to run out and buy our book just because you say 'nothing causes cancer?' A statement like that isn't going to help all the hundreds of thousands of cancer victims who will develop cancer this year."

"Excuse me, Carter," he said in alarm. "Your blood pressure is rising fast. And we're pumping out adrenalin and hormones like crazy in here. It's getting a little uncomfortable. Please simmer down."

"I'm *glad* you're uncomfortable, you insufferable microbe! I've spent a lot of time on this book on your say-so alone.

Now I find out that you don't know what you're talking about. I don't appreciate your making a fool of me."

"Would it make you feel better to find out that your best human scientists agree with me?"

"Fat chance. All our scientists agree that cancer is a family of over 250 different diseases. And they all say that literally thousands of chemicals cause cancer. There are over two thousand chemicals in cigarette smoke alone, and many of them are known to cause cancer."

"Okay, Carter. Cool down. Besides the T lymphocytes of your immune defense forces, who knows more about cancer than anyone else?"

"I guess that would have to be the National Cancer Institute and the American Cancer Society."

"Do you by any chance have a copy of *The American Cancer Society Cancer Book* handy? If I read your memory correctly, it was published by Doubleday & Company in 1986."

"Sure, I have it right here."

"Good. Please turn to the Introduction and find page xix. On the third line down, begin reading with the word 'Only.' "

"All right, It says:

'Only when the immune system is incapable of
destroying these malignant cells will cancer develop.' "

"Right. Now, Carter, tell me in your own words exactly what you just read."

"As long as you cells of my immune system are doing your job the way you're supposed to, I will never get cancer."

"Finally! You got the message and you do understand. Let's review what I've taught you so far."

"But that was only one sentence. . ."

"Okay. Read the next sentence."

"Here goes:'

'This theory has been bolstered by what happens
when the immune system breaks down, as it does
in patients with AIDS (Acquired Immune Deficiency

Syndrome). Several rare types of cancer, such as Karposi's sarcoma, Burkitt's lymphoma, and chronic myeloid leukemia, are common among AIDS victims. More recently, other cancers have been noted as well.'

"I see your point, Larry. Let's review."

"Okay, Carter. What can cause a cell to mutate?"

"Anything and everything, even bad luck," I answered.

"You could say that."

"I just did."

"Enough banter. How many times does a cell have to mutate before it can begin to qualify as a potential cancer cell?" he quizzed.

"At least twice."

"What's the difference between the terms carcinogenic and mutagenic?" he asked.

"Nothing," I answered promptly.

"Right again. And what's the most damage any chemical classified as a carcinogen can do?"

"It can cause a cell to mutate twice."

"Possible, but not probable. Remember, the odds are stacked in favor of my house, your body. The final question: What causes cancer?"

"Nothing. An inefficient immune system allows cancer to develop."

"That wasn't so hard was it? The most promising approach to cancer therapy lies within your own body. Instead of poisoning the body, as many conventional therapies do, wouldn't it be better to boost your body's own defenses against cancer? If you humans beef up your immune system, cancer cells won't stand a chance. We'll get 'em before they can cause any trouble. And, if you want to do something really important, find out how and why cells go wrong and turn into mutations in the first place. All you humans live out your entire lives with mutant cells roaming around inside your bodies.

"So far, Carter, we have identified mutant cells and have determined that there are definable differences between mutations and cancer. But we still have to identify exactly what cancer is and how it reacts."

"Good idea, Larry. Every reference to cancer I've found indicates that cancer is a family of over one hundred diseases. What do you say to that?"

"All cancers are colonies of disobedient cells, cells which disobey the laws of the body. These laws are known as negative feedback controls."

"Are you saying that cancer is only one disease, rather than a whole related family of diseases?" I asked.

"At the risk of repeating the obvious I remind you for the umpteenth time that *cancer is not a disease*. Cancer is a symptom of an inefficient immune system, a red-flag signifying that the immune defense forces are falling down on the job."

"Don't get hot under the collar, Larry."

"I don't wear a collar, Carter."

"How do you explain the many different types of cancer?"

"I can understand how even your best cancer specialists are still confused about what cancer is and what it isn't," he said sympathetically. "All cancers are colonies of uncontrolled cells which ignore the laws of the body. But, because a cancer cell arises from a normal cell, it takes on the basic characteristics of the normal tissue it calls home. For example, if the original cell comes from normally slow-growing tissue, the malignant cell will be slow-growing. If malignant cells develop from fast-growing tissue, that cancer colony will grow rapidly."

"So, because skin cells are constantly replacing sloughed-off dead skin cells, skin cancer grows fast?" I asked, trying to understand the logic behind his explanation.

"Exactly. And the appearance of skin cancer cells is much different than, for instance, bone cancer cells. Although all the cells of your body carry the very same DNA blueprint which was established at the moment of conception, the cells are organized into more than 200 different families of cell tissue. And, because all cells can mutate, it is possible for cancer to wear 200 different disguises."

"I get it!" I exclaimed, as I began to see the big picture. "Back when our scientists began to classify various cancers, they categorized each one by the way it looked and acted. It's only logical that they would end up with hundreds of what they thought were entirely different cancers."

"Not only that," Larry continued, "because the transformation of a normal cell into a cancer cell is associated with the process of cell division, tissues that relinquish the capacity to divide, such as nerve cells, cells of the voluntary muscles, and even heart-muscle cells are virtually immune to cancer."

"Wow!" I exclaimed. "That's really interesting. But what makes cancer so dangerous?"

"As a cancer grows, it interferes with the functioning of the healthy tissue that surrounds it."

"That's usually when a person first discovers a lump, right?"

"Sure. As a cancer grows and causes pain, you humans start looking for the cause of the pain and may find a lump. But many cancers are not painful for a very long time," he cautioned.

"That's why so many cancers go undetected for so long."

"Undetected by you humans," he corrected. "We know immediately. The T cells identify each cancer cell long before it becomes a threat to your life and health. We immediately begin to build an army to combat each colony. As a matter of fact, Carter, most humans never know about more than 95 percent of all the cancer colonies in their bodies. The only ones you humans know about are the ones that overwhelm the immune defense forces."

"How can we keep that from happening, Larry?"

"I'll explain about that later on in the book, Carter. For the purpose of this chapter, let's stick to the subject and continue to identify the characteristics of cancer."

"Okay," I agreed. "Cancer spreads. How does this happen?"

"Not all cancer cells spread, or *metastasize* as your scientists term it. You have to remember that cancer cells are renegades. They not only disobey growth limits, they don't even become very attached to each other. So it's easy for some of the cells from a primary cancer to break away and move to another part of the body where they proceed to set up camp. If metastasis does occur, the cells from a malignant tumor move from one part of the body to another. And they start a new colony, which your scientists call a 'secondary' cancer, wherever a tumor cell takes root."

"Which cancer is the most dangerous?"

"It all depends on where they are located. But secondary cancers are just as dangerous as primary cancers."

"Why?"

"Let's look at what happens. When a tumor begins growing in bone, for example, it weakens your structural strength considerably. Even a normal amount of physical pressure might cause an affected bone to snap. Or, when a cancer colonizes the brain, lungs, or liver, all highly susceptible to wandering cells because of the large volume of blood which flows through them at all times, the growth can interfere with essential life support systems."

"It's easy to see that problems can develop wherever a tumor plants itself. In one sense, whether it is malignant or benign isn't important. As it grows and pushes into normal tissue, size becomes a factor."

"That's right, Carter. Also, of the more than 200 types of normal cells, a proportion of them are hormone-producing organ cells. If cancer occurs in these important cells, the cellular mechanism which controls the production of certain chemicals is thrown out of whack. The danger here is that certain chemicals which the body needs can't be produced, and others may be overproduced. Either way, the vital chemical balance of the body goes out of control."

"Can you be a little more specific, Larry?"

"Sure. For example, a tumor in the testes might stimulate the production of enough female hormones to cause a male to develop breasts and even a pregnancy test can come back positive in the male so affected. And tumors of the female ovaries have been known to secrete so much of the male hormone *testosterone* that some unfortunate women have developed facial hair that mimics a beard."

"Those effects could really mess up a social life," I remarked.

"That's the least of their worries," he shot back tartly. "Because the DNA of every normal cell in the body has all of the information it needs to function as any other cell of the body, a mutated cell can take over the responsibilities of any other cell. For example, certain types of lung cancer have been known to produce the hormones that are normally produced in the pituitary gland, causing dangerously high blood pressure, serious kidney disorders, and even weakening muscle structure."

"Larry, I think what you're telling me is that virtually any symptom, anything from a skin rash to an hallucination, might conceivably signify a tumor playing games inside the body."

"Yes, that's quite true, Carter. Even a general feeling of malaise, the appearance of not being quite up to snuff, and an unexplained weight loss can actually turn out to be major symptoms of early cancer."

"Why is it that people with cancer are always so weak?"

"Because cancer cells proliferate so rapidly, tumors appropriate a lot of the body's energy. Cancer cells greedily absorb nutrients at the expense of normal cells. The tumors grow strong, as the human grows weak."

"You've taught me a lot, Larry. To be fair to our hard-working scientists and medical doctors, I have to point out that it's easy to understand the confusion they've been laboring under for so long. Cancer has so many faces, personalities, sizes and growth patterns, and hides in such a wide variety of symptoms, that it's no wonder even the best minds in the country don't have a firm fix on cancer yet."

"Unfortunately, Carter," he said sadly, "you humans will continue to die of cancer as long as your scientists treat it as a disease. You see, I'm afraid they'll keep on looking for a 'magic bullet' that doesn't exist . . . or a super vaccine that will conquer cancer the same way vaccinations eliminated polio, mumps, chicken pox, and smallpox. In the meantime, it's scary to know that your medical experts will continue to cut, radiate, or poison already weakened bodies with chemotherapeutic chemicals in their misguided effort to fight against a foe they have yet to properly identify."

"I suppose you have a better solution."

"Carter, I have the only real answer to cancer. The cells that finally do transform themselves into viable cancer cells have such a battle before them from an army of such incredible magnitude that it makes me proud to be a part of it. You humans just don't seem to understand how efficient your immune defense forces really are, and how fast the system can be expanded under emergency conditions."

"Tell me."

"Tomorrow. You didn't hear the alarm sounding, but I'm being paged. I'm needed elsewhere right now and, if you know what's good for you, you'll wish me 'bon voyage.' "

"What's going on?," I asked anxiously. "Am I in trouble?"

"Not if I get there in time."

"Godspeed, Larry."

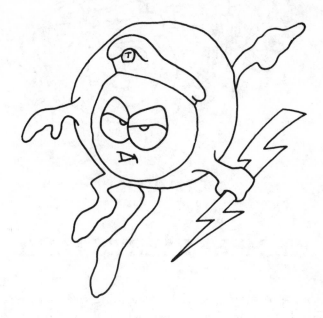

Bibliography

Holleb, AI, MD (ed): The American Cancer Society Cancer Book. Garden City, New York: Doubleday and Co, 1986.

Smedley, H, Sikora, K and Stephney, R: Cancer, What It Is and How It's Treated. Oxford, Great Britian: Basil Blackwell Ltd, 1985.

Winter, R: Cancer Causing Agents. New York: Crown Publishers Inc, 1979.

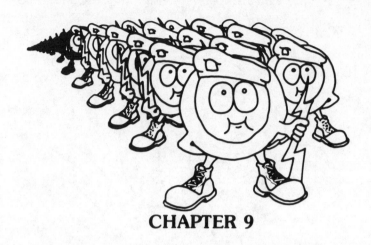

CHAPTER 9

WE MEET LARRY'S FAMILY

"Good morning, Larry. Is everything okay in there?"

"Good morning, Carter. Yes, all A-OK, as your astronauts say."

"Thanks for the good work, my friend. I'm sitting here in front of my word processor with my mind as blank as I can make it. I've been thinking about all those preconceived notions you told me were wrong. I did go back and review some medical books and I think . . . No, I *know* we're onto something big here."

"You got that right! By the way, Carter, I enjoyed your exercise session this morning. It was very stimulating. What do you call it?"

"The exercise?"

"Yes."

"It's called rebounding. You might have noticed that I do it every morning."

"Yes, I have noticed. And because of your 'rebounding,' as you call it, I am much stronger. You might be interested to know that my buddies and I are able to make rounds much faster when you rebound in the morning. Thanks for the boost."

"My pleasure, Larry. I'm glad to know it helps."

"To work, Carter. Let's begin by discussing what you found in the medical books."

"Well, I found some interesting stuff in the Seventh Edition of the *Textbook of Medical Physiology* authored by Dr. Arthur C. Guyton. Chapter 31 discusses the lymphatic system. On page 361, it says:

'The lymphatic system represents an accessory route by which fluids can flow from the interstitial spaces into the blood. And, most important of all, the lymphatics can carry proteins and large particulate matter away from the tissue spaces, neither of which can be removed by absorption directly into the blood capillary. We shall see that the removal of proteins from the interstitial spaces is an absolutely essential function, without which we would die within 24 hours.' "

"And what did you make of that, Carter?"

"The way I see it, Larry, there are two things we can do with that paragraph."

"Like what?"

"We can accept it at face value, or simply brush it off by saying that Dr. Guyton doesn't know what he's talking about."

"What do you think we should do?"

"If we accept it at face value, then we have an obligation to find out all we can about the lymphatic system."

"Why?"

"According to Dr. Guyton, if the lymphatic system shuts down for just 24 hours, we die."

"Is that important to you?"

"You bet it is! It's also important to my family."

"I'm glad you feel that way."

"Why?"

"Because I also feel you should know all you can about your lymphatic system, because our very lives depend on it... yours *and* mine."

"Okay, Larry, that's clear. But if the lymphatic system is so important, why don't we know more about it?"

"Is it taught in your schools?"

"No. I didn't even know what the lymphatic system looks like until you took me on that whirlwind tour the other day. My research included the study of numerous books written by scientific and medical authorities, but these books are not read by the average person. They are hard to read because they are written in medical terminology."

"What you're saying is that the information covering the lymphatic system is available to medical authorities?"

"Certainly. It must be, because that's where I found it. It's amazing what the general public doesn't know about how to keep well. In fact, it's beginning to worry me."

"Are you aware that nearly 60 percent of your total body weight is water? And that one-third of your body fluid is extracellular, meaning that it's outside the cells?"

"I really never thought much about it, Larry. Like most people, I always assumed that most of my body fluid is blood. I remember the old saying: 'Man is made of muscle and blood, skin and bones; a mind that's weak and a back that's strong.' "

"That's because nobody talks about the lymph fluid, Carter. But only 12 percent of your body fluid is blood, and 62 percent of your bodily fluid is inside the cells. What that means is that 36 percent of your fluid is lymph."

"Wow!" I exclaimed. "There's three times more lymph fluid in the body than blood!"

"Right. And another name for lymph fluid is water. The lymph is the fluid that surrounds all the cells. It is the cell's environment."

"Are all of you cells surrounded by water?"

"No. Not all of us. The bone cells are surrounded by bone minerals. But all cells depend directly on extracellular water for food. Even bone cells are fed by the lymph fluid through minute channels. Lymph is filled with nutrients on their way to the cells, waste products thrown off by the cells, hormones, and enzymes. Leukocytes, lymphocytes, monocytes, antibodies, and other white blood cells are able to travel wherever water exists."

"As a lymphocyte, that means you can travel throughout the entire body."

"Sure. And just as the air around humans is in motion constantly, the lymph fluid that surrounds the cells is also in contant motion."

"Just as it's refreshing for a human to experience a fresh breeze in a stuffy, polluted room . . ."

"You're on the right track. We cells are able to function better with fresh lymph fluid filled with the proper concentrations of oxygen, glucose, and all other nutrients. When fresh supplies replace the waste products of cells, the toxins, bacteria, viruses, poisons, trash and debris, we cells are healthier, and so are you."

"If the lymph fluid is the environment of the cell and the lymph is in constant motion, what causes the lymph to circulate? Everyone knows that the heart pumps blood through the arteries, lungs, capillaries, and veins. I've seen pictures of the heart, and I can feel it beat inside me. But how does lymph circulate?"

"The answer to that is also found on page 361."

"What?"

"Don't forget that whatever you read is available to me also," he reminded me. "You were reading *Medical Physiology* . . ."

"Yes. Here it is in big bold print:
'THE LYMPHATIC PUMP. Valves exist in all lymph
channels. In the large lymphatics, valves exist *every
few millimeters,* and in the smaller lymphatics, the
valves are much closer than this. Motion pictures of
exposed lymph vessels in animals and human beings

show that when a lymph vessel becomes stretched with fluid, the smooth muscles in the wall of the vessel automatically contract. Furthermore, each segment of the lymph vessel between successive valves functions as a separate automatic pump. That is, the filling of a segment causes it to contract and the fluid is pumped through the valve to the following lymphatic segment. This fills the subsequent segment and a few second later, it too contracts. The process continues all along the lymphatic system until the fluid is finally emptied back into the blood stream from the thoracic duct into the vena cava right underneath the collar bones.' "

"You see, Carter, the heart is on automatic. It starts beating before you are born and continues to beat until you die. But the lymphatic system is completely dependent on some kind of movement to stimulate the pumping action. Please continue reading."

"I'm fascinated, Larry. Here goes:

'In addition to the intrinsic contractions of the lymph vessel walls, there are other factors which cause the lymph pump to function. Almost anything that compresses the lymph vessel can also cause pumping, such as the contraction of a muscle, movements of body parts, arterial pulsations, and even a body massage. Obviously, the lymphatic pump becomes very active during exercise, often increasing lymph flow as much as ten to thirty-fold. On the other hand, during periods of rest, lymph flow is very sluggish.' "

"Let me give you an example, Carter. While you were rebounding this morning, your lymphatic system was moving about twenty times as fast as it is right now. That's why it's so easy to keep you healthy when you rebound regularly. Thank you."

"No, Larry. I should thank you. You and all of my other lymphocytes. Is there anything else I can do to make your job easier?"

"Plenty, but we'll get into all that later on. I want you to understand everything there is to know about your lymphatic system first."

"Okay. Tell me about the lymph tubes."

"You mean the veins?"

"Yes."

"The lymphatic system consists of millions of lymph veins. The smaller ones have walls just one cell thick, but the thoracic duct, the largest lymph vein, is as big as your thumb."

"Sort of like the cardiovascular system."

"The lymphatic system is different from the cardiovascular system. Your cardiovascular network is a closed-circuit system made up of arteries, capillaries, veins, and the heart. Your lymphatic system works more like an internal vacuum-cleaning system. The lymphatic terminals feed into the lymph veins. Surely you remember that from the tour."

"Oh, yes. The vacuum-cleaner nozzle things. But they don't suck up dirt and air, they suck up water and metabolic waste."

"You've got the idea. The minute quantity of fluid that returns to the circulatory system by way of the lymphatics is extremely important. Substances of high molecular weight, such as proteins, can't be reabsorbed into the veins of the cardiovascular system through the capillaries, but can flow into the lymphatic capillaries almost completely unimpeded."

"Why is that?"

"The lymphatic terminals are made up of endothelial cells attached by anchoring filaments to the connective tissue between the surrounding tissue cells. The edge of one cell usually overlaps the edge of another one, leaving it free to flap inward. These minute valves allow metabolic trash and debris into the lymphatic terminal, but prevent it from escaping."

"Now please put that in terms I can understand."

"Easy. Large particles of dead cells, viruses, and trash can be sucked into the lymphatic terminals along with the excess water. But it's a one-way street. The junk can't get out again."

"Where does all that extracellular fluid come from?"

"It escapes from the capillaries of the cardiovascular system. See, Carter, the capillaries are like strainers. They're filled with little sieve-like holes which allow oxygen, nutrients, and protein molecules to escape into the tissue spaces. But the holes are too small to permit red blood cells to flow out of the cardiovascular system. That's why blood doesn't surround the cells, as lymph fluid does. After delivering its life-giving oxygen and nutrients to the cells, 90 percent of the fluid is reabsorbed at the venal end of the capillaries through the same minute holes. Only 10 percent of the fluid that escapes from the capillaries actually moves through the lymphatic system."

"You said red blood cells are too large to fit through the tiny holes in the capillaries. How do you white blood cells get out?"

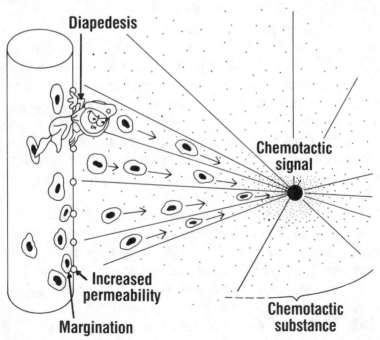

"We're tricky. We have the ability to change our shapes when necessary. I simply stick a pseudopodium through..."

"A 'what?' "

"A *pseudopodium*. That's part of my ectoplasm, my skin, my outside surface. Oh, just think of it as an arm, Carter."

"Okay," I said agreeably. "What is it you do with your pseudopodium?"

"I squeeze a pseudopodium through a tiny pore in the capillary about one-tenth my size and ooze in. That's the way we white blood cells get out of your blood stream when the red blood cells cannot."

"So the red blood cells don't have your ability to squeeze through small spaces. You'd make a great cat burglar, Larry."

"A 'what?' "

"Never mind. Let's continue. The lymphatic system might have several nicknames then, depending on the background of the person describing it. It might be called the 'auxiliary circulatory system,' the 'garbage collector of the body,' the 'vacuum-cleaning system,' or even the 'immune system.' Each one of these names is descriptive of a particular function of the lymphatic system. Do you agree?"

"I guess so."

"Essentially, no particulate matter that enters the tissues can be absorbed directly into the capillary membranes because the sieve-like holes are too tiny. If the particles are not gobbled up locally in the tissues by the giant macrophages, they enter the lymph and flow through the lymphatic vessels into the lymph nodes, which are strategically located along the course of the lymphatic system."

"Are the lymph nodes those little nodules that swell up under the chin, in my groin, and under my arms when I get sick?" I asked.

"Right. You remembered! The nodes swell up because foreign particles are trapped there in a meshwork of tiny chambers. The chambers are populated with large numbers of those beneficent beasts, the macrophages, all waiting to eat the aliens and prevent them from general dissemination throughout your body.

"See, Carter," he explained, "your body is constantly exposed to bacteria, viruses, fungi, and parasites. These aliens cover your skin, are in your mouth, your lungs, and your nose. They live in your digestive system and even in the membranes lining your eyes. Many of these enemies of the body are capable of causing serious, sometimes fatal, damage if they are allowed to invade the deeper tissues and organs of the body. You are also exposed intermittently to other highly-infectious bacteria and viruses, on top of those which are normally present in your body. Some have the potential to cause a deadly disease, such as pneumonia, streptococcal infections, or typhoid fever."

"You're scaring me, Larry. What if an invading organism does succeed in entering the general circulation?"

"There still remain other lines of defense. The spleen functions a bit like the lymph nodes, except that its fluid is blood, not lymphatic fluid. The spleen permits red blood cells to squeeze through its meshwork, but abnormal red blood cells, metabolic trash, and debris are subject to immediate *phagocytosis*, meaning that they are eaten by the macrophages of the spleen."

"That's teriffic," I enthused. "As long as all of you guys are doing your job, I really don't have to worry about getting sick, do I?"

"You are absolutely right. You must realize by now, Carter, that the 'War on Cancer' declared by your government back in 1971 has to be fought inside the body. Problems can spring up in your cardiovascular system, your musculoskeletal system, your hard head, or your lymphatic system. There's a lot of places for the aliens to dig in. When the enemy shows one of its nasty faces, all the cells of your body become involved in the fight, either directly or indirectly. Depending on the outcome of the battle within, all the cells share in the sweet taste of victory, or the agony of defeat. We're all in this together, Carter."

"Larry, our scientists have the ability to extract blood or lymph fluid from the human body, prepare a slide, and look at the white blood cells under a microscope. I've seen video films that show the activity of you white blood cells as you destroy bacteria, viruses, and even cancer cells. But most of our readers don't have access to a microscope and will never see a video film of the battle. How can we help them understand what we're talking about here?"

"That shouldn't slow us down any, Carter. You see, there are two ways to 'see' anything. The first, of course, is to actually see it and experience it. The second way is to 'visualize' it with the aid of your imagination."

"Okay, Larry. Then our job is to activate the imagination of our readers. If we do our respective parts as co-authors well, we can show all the complex intrigue of what you call the battle within that's going on constantly in each of our readers at any given moment.

"I remember seeing the movie *The Longest Day* in which the major participants and the actual armies involved in preparation for the 'D Day' of World War II were visited by actors and cameras. Viewers were led step-by-step through the sequential happenings on that day which led up to the landing of the allied forces in Europe.

"In a previous chapter, Larry, you introduced our readers to the enemy, cancer. You explained that cancer is elusive and has many faces and told us why cancer is so confusing that the best medical authorities call it '. . . one of the supreme mysteries.' You even treated us to a cell's-eye view of your battlefield in a chapter of this book that I entitled 'The Larry Lymphocyte Guided Tour.' "

"There's still more to learn, Carter. I remind you that in 1971 when the U.S. declared war on cancer, your scientists still hadn't identified the immune defense force army which was already fighting that particular war, along with many others. I'm going to introduce you to an awesome army, a fantastic, ferocious fighting force, a search and destroy strike force so well organized that the chase scenes of those James Bond movies you like so much pale by comparison."

"That's quite a bold statement, Larry."

"Okay, Carter. I take that as a personal challenge. Let's compare fighting forces. Tell me about your army."

"You mean the United States armed forces?"

"Sure."

"Well, our armed forces include several branches, including the Army, Navy, Marines, and Air Force."

"Is that all?"

"No, of course not. There are several other branches, including the CIA, the reserves. . ."

"I get the picture, Carter. Just as your U.S. government has a complex protection system, your body has a special and very complex protection system for combating all the enemies of your body, foreign and domestic. This internal army is well equipped with the right ammunition. Ammunition, I might add, that's well beyond your latest scientific and medical technologies."

"The U.S. army is equipped with ships, boats, planes, tanks, submachine guns, secret agents, spies, foot soldiers, cavalrymen, gun boats, land mines, rifles and more."

"The army within puts your U.S. defense systems to shame," he said with pride.

"That statement needs some explanation."

"Right. The leukocytes, your white blood cells, are the mobile units of this microscopic army. We leukocytes are capable of traveling anywhere in your entire body as the need arises."

"Do all you guys look alike?"

"Well, there's a definite family resemblance, but there are six general types of leukocytes. Some of us are large, and others are very small. There's a lot of some of us, but others have very specialized responsibilities and are few in number."

"Where do all the white blood cells come from?"

"Some leukocytes are manufactured in the bone marrow, while others are manufactured in the lymphatic system, including the nodes, spleen, tonsils, and thymus."

"Wow! If leukocytes are manufactured in the bone marrow, how do they get through bone and into the rest of the body? Bones are awfully hard."

"All bones have built-in blood channels. All you need to remember is that all white blood cells are deployed either through the rapidly moving bloodstream, or the slower moving lymphatic pathways to wherever the body needs our protection."

"Just how big is this army we're discussing anyway?"

"In human terms, the forces of your immune defense system equal a standing army of close to two and one-half million men, 2,400,000 to be exact. And all of us are superbly armed and trained even more exactingly than those spectacular human commandos you call the Green Berets. Carter, your microscopic army is not only ready to fight all your enemies immediately, we've been defending your very life since before you were born. I also might add that we haven't received the credit due us for performing such a vital service. And we're not supported by tax dollars either," he remarked, in a bit of a huff. "We're an all-volunteer army. We accept our jobs as our solemn duty. Each member of your immune defense forces is ready to go wherever danger lurks. We fight for your life to the death without a moment's hesitation and without a thought for our own survival."

"An army of almost two and one-half million cells swarming around inside my body! That's incredible, Larry. How did you arrive at that figure anyway?"

"Leukocytes make up one percent of all the cells in your body. I read in your memory banks that the population of the U.S. is around 240 million people, Carter. And one percent of 240 million is 2,400,000. Incidentally, taken all together, our total weight comes to about two pounds per person."

"Perhaps this would be a good time for you to explain some of the individual responsibilities for the different divisions of this army."

"I will, Carter. But to keep things simple for you humans, I'm only going to describe the capabilities and responsibilities of just a few divisions of your magnificent fighting forces."

"Will you also identify them for us, Larry?"

"Certainly. More than half of the leukocytes in your body are made up of very efficient *polymorphonuclear neutrophils.* I'll call them neutrophils, for short. These fast-acting little guys attack and destroy invading bacteria, viruses, or other foreign agents by eating them up. The neutrophils are dedicated to one goal. They search out and destroy anything that might be harmful to the body."

"Do the neutrophils travel in the blood?"

"They stay in the bloodstream for just a few hours. Because they have the ability to dramatically change their shape, they're able to squeeze through. Even though the pores of the blood vessels are incredibly minute and the neutrophils are much bigger, they can constrict themselves and slide through a pore a bit at a time, much as a thread slips through the eye of a needle. And the neutrophils have the ability to move by themselves. Although red blood cells are pushed around by the flow of plasma in the cardiovascular system, the neutrophils travel alone. This capability is scientifically known as *ameboid motion*," he added.

"How fast do the neutrophils move?" I asked curiously.

"They can move several times their length in about a minute. More importantly, neutrophils have the ability to 'taxi' toward or away from the source of a chemical. This phenomenon is called *chemotaxis*. Because bacteria, toxins, and even the degenerated products of injured tissue create a chemical environment readily identified by neutrophils as a chemotoxic signal, vast hordes of leukocytes move from the capillaries into the injured and inflamed area to clean it up."

"Then this is what is known as 'inflammation,' " I mused.

"Right. When an inflammation occurs, within just a few short hours the number of neutrophils in the blood increases by four or five times, up to as many as 25,000 per cubic millimeter. Perhaps the most important weapon of the neutrophils is their ability to eat, or phagocytize, an invader."

"That means they don't stop working for lunch," I observed with a smile.

"Another talent of the leukocytes that should be called to your attention is their ability to identify the material they eat. If they didn't have this special capability, normal cells would be gobbled up as well."

"How can the neutrophils tell the good guys from the bad guys?" I asked

"Each healthy cell of the body carries an identification badge known as an *epitope*. The epitope is made up of very specific protein molecules which are easily read by the neutrophils. Cells wear their identification epitopes on the outside. When the badge information isn't exactly right, the neutrophils identify that cell as a foreigner, mutant, or traitor and carry out immediate destruction by ingestion."

"Let's see if I have this straight, Larry. Neutrophils are manufactured in the bone marrow and are then released into the bloodstream. They patrol the bloodstream for between four to eight hours, then squeeze out through the pores of the capillaries. After that, the neutrophils spend the next four or five days roaming around searching the tissues for alien bacteria. What happens when they find infection someplace in the body?"

"In times of serious tissue infection, the neutrophil's entire lifespan can be compressed into just a few hours. They proceed rapidly to the affected area, ingest the invading organisms, and in the process are destroyed themselves."

"Poor little guys! How are they destroyed?"

"They don't know when to stop eating. As long as there is foreign matter in your body, they literally continue to eat until they explode."

"That's what I call real dedication."

"All your immune system defense forces are equally dedicated, Carter. When neutrophils and macrophages engage the enemy, large numbers of neutrophils and macrophages die, but not before they have destroyed large colonies of bacteria. The debris of dead soldier cells and dead bacteria on both sides is commonly known as pus. Pus formation continues to build until all infection is suppressed. If the infection is close to the outside of the body, the pus forms into a boil or blister and is eventually eliminated that way. If the infection is deep within the body, the debris is usually absorbed into the surrounding tissue.

"We'll talk more about the neutrophils when I tell you about a pitched battle between your defense forces and a cancer colony. But now that you've been intimately acquainted with the capabilities of the neutrophils, you'll be better able to understand the other arms of your crack fighting forces."

"That's fair, Larry. Please continue."

"Do you remember 'Jaws,' that magnificent old macrophage I pointed out to you awhile back?"

"Of course. He's really something."

"You bet he is. Jaws was born in the bone marrow as a tiny monocyte. After receiving a chemical danger signal, the bone marrow goes to work and produces an increased number of monocytes. Within just eight to twelve hours of manufacture, these tiny cells change from immature mites incapable of ingesting anything into fully mature macrophages. The macrophages have awesome powers, including the ability to move independently throughout the body toward an on-going battle."

"Are you saying that the monocytes and the macrophages

are one and the same cell, Larry? How can that be?" I asked incredulously.

"Few of your human scientists understand this either, Carter. The monocytes are very interesting. They make up only five percent of the white blood cells while in the bloodstream. But the only reason they hitch a ride in that great freeway is because that's the route they must travel from the bone marrow where they are formed into the tissue spaces where they are desperately needed.

"While the monocytes are in the bloodstream, they are young, immature, and incapable of fighting off a foreign invader. But once they slide through a capillary pore and emerge into the tissue spaces, the germs and bacteria better watch out! They immediately begin to expand to five times their birth size and are then known as macrophages."

"Even the name sounds big," I observed.

"And they live up to their name, too," Larry said earnestly. "Macrophages are devastating to the enemy. They have all the talents and capabilities of the neutrophils, and then some. Where a neutrophil can eat between five and twenty bacteria before it dies of its magnificent protective gluttony, the macrophage has the capability of phagocytizing as many as one hundred of the ugly things. When necessary, the giant macrophages can even gobble up the whole red blood cells that have gone wrong, malarial parasites, and even dead neutrophils who have given their lives to the cause."

"And after the macrophages have eaten their fill, do they also have to die?" The thought made me sad, somehow.

"No, not always," Larry assured me. "The macrophages have the extraordinary ability to excrete the residue of the digested enemies they eat. Macrophages are able to continue destroying alien invaders for weeks, months, even years, before they die a natural death of old age."

"There's one thing I don't understand, Larry. If the macrophages are five times bigger than the neutrophils, how do they get around?"

"Although these giants have the ability to travel when an emergency signal galvanizes them into action, they usually attach themselves to various organs and tissues of the body. In a healthy, clean body - such as yours, Carter - the macrophages might spend the rest of their lives just guarding that particular part of the body from harm."

"Do all macrophages look and act alike, Larry?"

"Not really. The macrophages based in various tissues differ in appearance and action because of the differences in their respective environments. That's why your scientists are confused. When you humans began to study various organs and found macrophages in residence, they mistook them for different varieties of cells."

"Hmmm. It sounds to me as if they used the same method of classification that they used for cancer."

"That's right. They even gave the macrophages different names. Your scientists call the macrophages in the liver *Kupffer's cells*; in the lungs they are known as *alveolar* macrophages; in the subcutaneous tissues they are called *histiocytes* and *clasmatocytes*; and in the brain they are dubbed *microglia*. But they are all macrophages, and perform the same functions in the same way as all macrophages."

"That is interesting," I mused.

"Okay, Carter. You've just been introduced to the neutrophils, monocytes, and macrophages. I'll stage a mock battle for you a little later on."

"What about you, Larry? Are you a neutrophil or a macrophage?"

"Neither. I thought I had made that clear earlier, Carter. I am a T Lymphocyte. More specifically, I'm a cytotoxic T cell."

"You make that sound very important."

"You bet your life. It is important. Without us lymphocytes, your life would be very short and you'd be sick all the time. You could have mumps more than once, and measle germs would visit you often."

"All right already. Teach me about lymphocytes. I'm sorry. I didn't mean to get your dander up."

"I don't have dander."

"Ahem, right. Getting back to business... I thought the terms lymphocytes, leukocytes, and white blood cells were interchangeable... that all you guys were one and the same."

"That's how much you know about your immune system."

"I always assumed the lymphatic system was named after you lymphocytes," I said logically. "Is it possible it was misnamed?"

"So what else is new?" he answered in derision. "Even cancer was named after the crab, a lifeform that has nothing to do with the body. At least we lymphocytes live in the lymphatic system... and in the lymph nodes, tonsils, adenoids, spleen, appendix, and many other areas as well."

"Is that where you got your start?"

"I was created in the bone marrow, just as all other lymphocytes were. But before we matured, we were separated into two groups of lymphocytes and sent off to separate schools."

"Sent to school?" I asked incredulously.

"Don't act so pompous, Carter. Do you think humans are the only beings capable of learning? Even fish swim in schools. Yes. We were sent to school to learn our responsibilities."

"Where are these 'cell schools'?"

"Some of us lymphocytes are sent to the School of Thymus. That's where I went. When we graduate, we get our letters. That's why my cousins and I are known as T cells."

"And the T stands for 'thymus,' I suppose."

"Carter, sometimes you amaze me with your powers of deduction. Pure genius."

"You're not the only one who went to school, Larry," I said. "What did you learn at Thymus School?"

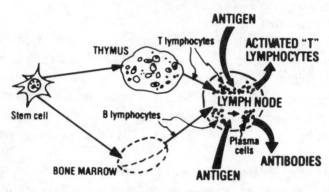

CELL-MEDIATED IMMUNITY

ANTIGEN

THYMUS

T lymphocytes

ACTIVATED "T" LYMPHOCYTES

Stem cell

B lymphocytes

LYMPH NODE

Plasma cells

ANTIBODIES

BONE MARROW

ANTIGEN

HUMORAL IMMUNITY

"Most of us T cell lymphocytes are taught how to identify and fight only one particular invader. As soon as we graduate, we are released from the thymus and sent into the bloodstream for a few hours. Then we 'Tees' find our way to one of the lymph nodes. Once in a node, we settle in and wait for the specific invader that we've been trained to kill. When one of those specific ugly aliens shows up, we do our duty right smartly and destroy the dirty enemy. Killing the alien activates our special programming. We then reproduce at a highly accelerated rate, forming tremendous numbers of duplicate lymphocytes which are known as sensitized T cells. The sensitized T cells are released into the lymph fluid and carried into the bloodstream. We circulate through all the tissue fluids and back to the lymph again, keeping a sharp eye peeled for invaders as we make our rounds. Sensitized T cells circulate around and around the circuit, sometimes for many years."

"That's very impressive, Larry. But you mentioned two groups of lymphocytes. What about the others?"

"The other group of lymphocytes go to Bone School and 'bone up' on how to produce a massive army of antibodies when a particular foreign substance is identified in the body. Can you guess what these lymphocytes are called?"

"B lymphocytes?"

"There! You did it again, Carter. Pure genius."

"I can't believe this," I muttered. "I'm being laughed at by a figment of myself."

Larry pretended not to hear and continued, "After graduation, the B cells are allowed to circulate freely in the blood for a few hours before they take up residence in the lymphoid tissue. There they sit and secretly await a specific invader. Each one of the B lymphocytes is capable of producing only one type of antibody, and can only be activated by one type of invader."

"And all of this 'educating' takes place in the thymus for the T cells, or the bones for the B cells?"

"Yes. Our respective educations have to be very exact. There are at least a million different types of B lymphocytes, and just as many of us T lymphocytes. All of us are capable of forming highly specific antibodies, or sensitized cells, when our programming is activated by the appropriate enemy."

"Is this how a person becomes immune to a particular disease?"

"Right. But immunity isn't acquired until an enemy alien arrives on the scene. The foreigner always has some chemical compound in its makeup that is different from any other compound of the cells that really belong to the body. Your scientists call this substance the *antigen*. The antigen is the equivalent of the foreign invader's secret code. All that's necessary is for the code to penetrate the lymphoid tissue in any part of the lymphatic system. Once that happens, we lymphocytes decipher the code and it's 'goodbye Charlie.' A standing army of antibodies and sensitized T cells are produced to fight off any alien with the same code that might dare to invade the body in the future."

"Are you a sensitized T cell, Larry?"

"You're getting close, Carter. There are three types of T cells. The T cell divisions include cytotoxic T cells, helper T cells, and suppressor T cells. We're all kissing cousins, but we do have our own responsibilities.

"I myself am a cytotoxic T cell," he explained proudly. "I am one of an army of millions of direct-attack cells of your immune defense forces, Carter. We're capable of killing almost any foreign invader. For this reason, we are frequently called killer cells."

"I'm not sure what you mean by 'cytotoxic,' Larry."

"We are known as cytotoxic cells, because we kill by poisoning the enemy," he explained.

"I see. The neutrophils and macrophages destroy my enemies by eating them. But your method of destruction is different then. You poison them. Is that right?"

"You got it. I only have to eat the ones I like, the tasty morsels. You humans have a saying that covers the situation: 'Love your enemies.' "

"That's not what that saying means, Larry. What poison do you use against the bad guys?"

"We use special substances called *lysosomol enzymes* that we manufacture ourselves. One of them is hydrogen peroxide."

"How do you get the enemy to take poison? Ask them to open their mouths?"

"They don't have mouths."

"I know. I was only joking."

"We simply embrace the enemy, hold him close, and inject the poison directly into the body of the invader. It doesn't take long," he said nonchalantly.

"Why do you use poison as a weapon, instead of eating them as the macrophages do?"

"Because when we kill an enemy with poison, rather than ingesting it, we can attack and kill many organisms, often without being harmed ourselves."

"That is exciting!" I enthused. "Would you say then that you cytotoxic T cells are the ultimate weapon of my immune defense forces?"

"No. Just the smartest. There is no 'ultimate weapon,' Carter. Each cell has responsibilities that it must fulfill in order to protect your body. It's all teamwork; there aren't any 'top guns' in here. I must tell you that we cytotoxic T cells are especially lethal to cancer cells, and that's good. But we create problems for your doctors, because we also attack the cells of transplanted organs or any other cells that are 'foreign' to the body."

"In other words, if I had a heart transplant, for example, the doctors would have to control your activity."

"Yes, but 'control' isn't correct. 'Kill' is the right term. That's what immunosuppressive drugs are used for when a person has an organ transplant, Carter."

"I hate to think about having my immune system put out of action, but I suppose there isn't any other choice. Sometimes the only chance for life we humans have is a transplanted donor organ to replace an organ of our own that no longer functions sufficiently to sustain life."

With all I had learned, the thought of being without the protection of my internal defenses was so frightening that I quickly changed the subject.

"Larry, the U.S. has a Distant Early Warning System known as the DEW line. It's made up of hundreds of radar stations that ceaselessly monitor the skies looking for any sign of an unfriendly invasion. You said awhile back that the immune system defenses were better than the federal defense systems of the nation. Do you and your buddies have an early warning system?"

"Of course. We have outposts strategically located that intercept enemy spies before they are allowed to enter the body. The lympoid tissue is our equivalent of your radar. For example, the tonsils intercept antigens that enter by way of the throat. The adenoids catch aliens trying to sneak in through the nose. And the lympoid tissue in your appendix and intestines guard against antigen invaders that hide in food."

"Larry, do you realize you've named many parts of the body that some surgeons still think of as unnecessary? Tonsils and adenoids used to be routinely removed, and many people have had their appendix or spleen taken out."

"Does that tell you how much your doctors knew about your immune system a few years back?" he asked scornfully. "To continue, the lympoid tissue of the spleen and bone marrow is able to decipher codes of the aliens that make it all the way to the blood. Lymphoid tissue is also located in the many lymph nodes throughout the body to identify a foreigner that might try to invade the tissue spaces."

"I see it would take several chapters to describe all the divisions of my ferocious internal fighting forces. However, because we are really only concerned about cancer in this book, let's talk about the cells you call 'traitors.'

"I've got something right here that might be interesting to you, Larry. Our doctors are beginning to give you credit. In his book *Nutrition Breakthrough*, Dr. Robert C. Atkins, M.D. begins his Chapter 17 on Cancer with these words:

" 'Doctors through the years have considered the immune system useful for fighting infectious organisms and in wound healing. Only recently have they begun to recognize that this very immune system can be useful for fighting off illnesses which have never been considered 'catching.' The most interesting is cancer.

" 'The matchup of what we know about our immunity with what we know about cancer holds out hope of providing answers we have all been seeking. The question raised is a tantalizing one: If the body's immune system helps control cancer, then is it not possible that the true breakthrough against cancer may be found in strengthening our immunity factors?' "

"You must have really had to search for that book for a long time, Carter. I'm afraid that most of your doctors and scientists are still a long way from understanding the relationship between your immune system and cancer."

"I agree with you, Larry. And so does Dr. Atkins. In Chapter 15, he writes:

" 'When I was a medical student, it took only a few days to learn all of what was known at that time about this defense system within our bodies. In the last few years, there has been a veritable explosion of information dealing with every facet of our immune system . . . We are now at the dramatic point where information (about the immune system) is being gathered. When it is fully developed, it will constitute one of the greatest medical breakthroughs. . .' "

"That's good to hear, Carter," Larry broke in. "And I must say that together we are making a substantial contribution to the growing body of knowledge that's being collected on the immune system. Would you like to hear about some of my first-hand experiences on the battlefield?"

"You bet!"

"Good. I love to reminisce. Put a fresh sheet of paper in your machine and get ready to start a new chapter. Let's title it *War Stories.*

Bibliography

Atkins, MD, RZ: Dr. Atkins' Nutrition Breakthrough. New York: William Morrow and Co, 1981.

Baram, P, et al (eds): Immunologic Tolerance and Macrophage Function. Holland: Elsevier/North, 1979.

Guyton, AC: Text Book of Medical Physiology. Philadelphia: WB Saunders Co, 1986.

Ham, AW, et al: Blood Cell Formation and the Cellular Basis of Immune Responses. Philidelphia: JB Lippincott Co, 1979.

Lancki, EW, et al: Cell Surface Structures Involved in T-Cell Activation. Immunol. Rev, 81:65 1984.

CHAPTER 10

WAR STORIES

"Okay, Larry. I'm ready. You must have had many life-threatening experiences in your career. Tell me one that stands out in your DNA."

"I'll tell you one that you didn't even know about, Carter. A mole smaller than a pinhead erupted in the middle of your back about six months ago. You didn't know about it, because you couldn't see it. The ugly thing began to develop right after you came home from your vacation on the beaches of Hawaii.

"Comparatively speaking, the cells of this mole were growing much faster than any other cells on your back. The rapid proliferation stimulated some of the nerve endings in the general area, and it began to itch. You scratched it along with the rest of your itchy back as your skin began to dry and flake. While you were basking in the hot Hawaiian sunshine, the top layer of your skin cells began to die from your sunburn, then tan, then burn again.

"As time went on, your itching and scratching activated my cousins, the macrophages, just under the surface of your skin. The macrophages recognized the unfamiliar proteins being produced by the darker cells and realized they were mutations.

118

Jaws and Big Mack and some of the others attacked the melanoma from underneath. Within a few days of your return home, all that was left was a small patch of dry skin that fell off in the shower. You continued living a very normal, happy, and carefree life and never knew you had skin cancer."

I was a little disappointed and let him know it. "Pooh, Larry, how can you call that a 'war story?' It doesn't even sound like much of a skirmish."

"You're right, Carter. And as long as I have anything to do with your immune defense forces, that's all any of our confrontations with enemy aliens will ever be."

"What if I were a smoker? What kind of war stories would you have to tell then?"

"Okay, let's set up a possible scenario. Let's say that you've been smoking since you were sixteen and know you should quit. You've been coughing more in the past two weeks than ever before. Lately you've noticed that when you cough up phlegm, it's a dark, sickening, foul smelling mucus. The lymph nodes in your groin, under your arms, under your chin, and around your neck are swollen. You've been feeling tired and lethargic. But, you tell yourself, that's the way a person is supposed to feel during the hot days of summer.

"Deep inside your lung are hundreds, perhaps thousands, of patches of scar tissue. These are signs of battles won by your immune system. But just two weeks ago, a new spot appeared in your lungs and it's being constantly aggravated. It bleeds, heals, and bleeds again because of the more than 2,000 chemicals in the cigarette smoke you inhale so greedily. Some of the rapidly-dividing cells have mutated for a second time, creating a strange new protein molecule that's not familiar to the macrophages in residence in your lungs. Several of them immediately attack and eat the mutating cells. They quickly capture the secret code of the mutant genes and pass it along to a neighboring neutrophil. The neutrophil slowly makes its way to the closest lymph node so that the antigen can be decoded.

"But, in the meantime, the small group of mutant cells begins to grow and grow until they weigh about one-hundredth of an ounce. The growing cancer colony ruptures a small blood vessel and, because cancer cells have a tendency to break away, many of them are washed into the bloodstream. It only takes five beats of your heart, Carter, for the blood to be pumped throughout your entire body. Metastasis happens quickly.

"Just a week ago, the cancer was sending almost a million mutant cells into your bloodstream every day. Because the blood is a particularly hostile environment to mutant cells, very few of these ugly traitors survived to establish colonies elsewhere. In fact, because of the antibodies the lymph nodes pour into the bloodstream, only about one out of every thousand cancer cells can survive more than two weeks.

"Three days ago, another colony of mutant cells broke away from your lungs, entered the bloodstream, and finally got caught in the sinuses of your liver. Nutrients are plentiful in the circulatory system of the liver, and the cancer was very comfortable there. The new colony was under siege by sensitized T cells and the macrophages of the liver, but the cancer continues to grow.

"Yesterday, your white blood count doubled because your lymph nodes are struggling valiantly to keep up and are pouring vast numbers of antibodies and T lymphocytes into your bloodstream. But this morning some of the mutant cells broke off from the cancer colony in your liver and spread throughout the rest of your body.

"By the end of next week, many small cancer colonies, each one no larger than a pinhead, will be dividing, multiplying, proliferating, stealing oxygen and nutrients from healthy cells, and creating havoc throughout your entire body.

"It's a very good thing that your immune system defense forces have already identified the mutant cells and are producing antibodies and sensitized T-cells to fight the traitors. As soon as a colony is established, the macrophages in the area phagocytize some of the mutant cells, thereby releasing the antigenic message which will activate the sensitized T-cells in the area. If the war goes according to plan, less than a month from the original eruption of cancerous tissue in your lungs, all the different cancer colonies which metastasized from the original will have been identified, isolated, and destroyed. All that's left then is for the cleanup crews to get busy.

"The macrophages and neutrophils residing in each area will eat up what's left of the dead cells who fell on each side of the battle. The lymphatic system will carry away some of the results of the carnage to the tonsils and adenoids. Your lymph nodes will swell and you'll have a sore throat. For the next few weeks, you'll notice whitish phlegm when you cough and spit, your throat will be scratchy and irritated, and your nose will run. You'll probably think you've caught a common cold, but your symptoms are the aftermath of a hard-fought battle. Unless you know better, you'll seek symptomatic relief and treat yourself with some over-the-counter chemicals designed to suppress the symptoms of a cold.

"In another week, your white blood count will drop back to normal. And, after the smoke of battle clears, you'll have minute scars throughout your entire body, plus new scar tissue in your lungs. Most of these scars will disappear in time. Your swollen lymph nodes will shrink... and you'll continue smoking.

"After all, it was just another bout of cancer that you didn't know about. And nobody but us cells will see the battle scars anyway."

"I don't know, Larry," I commented mildly. "In spite of all your dramatics, you just told me two stories that are impossible to verify."

"That's right, Carter. That's because most cancers you humans develop are never identified as cancer. How does a human know when he has cancer anyway?"

"When it's diagnosed by some medical doctor I guess."

"Are their methods of detection 100 percent accurate?"

"What do you mean?"

"Can your doctors find every cancer every time?"

"No. Some cancers go undetected for a long time."

"When do humans go to their doctors for this detection procedure?"

"When they suspect something's wrong, of course."

"Can you count on a human going to the doctor when they suspect something might be wrong?"

"No. Because they fear the unknown, some people stay away from doctors *especially* when they think something's gone wrong."

"Therefore, Carter," Larry said emphatically, "for the most part, the only cancers your doctors see are those which have been proliferating wildly out of control for weeks or months. These cancers are the ones which have grown big enough to be detected by some monitoring device, or which have caused enough problems to the host body to cause the victim to seek medical assistance.

"But what about all the cells which mutate twice and grow out of control for awhile, or even spread, until the immune system breaks the code, identifies the cancer, and builds a defense force large enough to destroy the colony? Is that verifiable, Carter?"

"No. Larry, you must realize that we can't base this whole book on your undoubted successes without verification. *I* believe you, little buddy. But the scientists and medical authorities won't accept your unsubstantiated word, you know."

"Who are we writing this book for, Carter? Human scientists and medical doctors have access to all the world's research and even have their own laboratories where they can prove or disprove any premise. They probably won't approve of our efforts anyway.

"What we are attempting to accomplish with this book is

to get the word out to the rest of the humans, those poor palookas who have been relying on their medical authorities for the right answers without getting 'em. You're a fairly knowledgeable human, Carter, but I have to tell you that I've been appalled at what even *you* don't know about keeping yourself well."

"Point well taken, Larry. But there's a mountain of published evidence out there which confirms every statement we've made in this book. For example, the David Salisbury story..."

"Tell it," he interrupted.

"I was just about to. Don't be so impatient and stop interrupting," I said testily. "David Salisbury of Astoria, Oregon was 29 years old when G.M. Boelling, M.D. found what he listed as 'a massive mediastinal and abdominal adenopathy.' Dr. Boelling's examination of David's abdomen on April 24th, 1980 showed 'a firm tender mass about the size of a volleyball in the left upper quadrant.' Dr. Boelling's educated guess that it was a lymphoma was confirmed by pathologists at St. John's Hospital in Longview, Washington. R.C. Harris, M.D. of that facility performed an exploratory operation on David called a *mediastimoscopy*, an operation used medically to permit a positive and expert identification of the problem.

"The exploratory operation revealed: 'The several irregular fragments of firm, pale gray tissue when viewed under the microscope verified that it was ... malignant lymphoma, nodular type.' "

"Carter, you have just described a runaway cancerous condition."

"I know, Larry, but listen to this: In a letter written to David on September 23, 1980, Dr. Boelling says, 'As you can see, the radiologist sees no evidence of a tumor remaining.' "

"Did David have surgery to remove the cancer?"

"No."

"Well, was he treated with radiation or chemotherapy?"

"No."

"Carter, are you telling me that a malignant lymphoma the size of a volleyball just disappeared without radiation, chemotherapy, or surgery... and that the disappearance of that really big mass of cancerous tissue was verified by medical doctors? Did the cancer come back later? Were David's records mixed up with a healthy person's?"

" 'No' to all of the above, Larry. The clincher was when Dr. Boelling of the Astoria Clinic wrote a 'To Whom It May Concern' letter for David Salisbury on May 14, 1985. After a complete physical examination, including laboratory studies, Dr. Boelling wrote: 'David is in excellent health and, specifically, there is no evidence of a malignancy.' "

"Whew! That is impressive, Carter. David certainly must have had an exceptionally strong and healthy immune system."

"Right. Now *that's* the kind of evidence I'm talking about, Larry. That's the kind of scientific documentation that impresses medical doctors and research scientists."

"Why didn't you say so, Carter?" he answered scornfully. "If that's all you want, you don't need me to supply it. There are over 200 well-documented cases of terminal cancer patients who have suddenly become cleared of cancer with no medical interference or scientific explanation. My stories were just for the purpose of making you aware of the literally millions of cancerous conditions which have never been detected or identified simply because the immune system defense forces functioned efficiently."

"Okay, Larry, simmer down. My next question is a simple one: Does the immune system have the ability to keep us healthy?"

"The answer is just as simple. *Yes*. As long as the immune system itself is healthy and functioning efficiently, the human will remain healthy and function efficiently."

"Terrific. But, I've got you now, Larry. . . If the forces of the immune defense system are as great as you like to think, why is it that cancer exists at all?"

"Think, human!" He let his aggravation show. "Virtually anything which reduces the efficiency of the immune defense forces will aid the enemy by creating an internal environment conducive to the proliferation of mutant cells. When you complicate our lives by making us defend against extraneous foreigners as well as the normal enemies of your body, including cancer, a cancer colony can grab the ball and run with it. That's when a colony grows large enough to be medically detected and your doctor says, 'You have cancer.'"

"That's really scary," I said. "Answer me two questions then, Larry."

"I'll try."

"First, what causes the immune system to break down enough to allow cancer? And, second, is it possible to restore the immune system defense forces after they're impaired?"

"Carter, those are the two most important questions in this whole book!"

"Oh? Why is that?"

"Because the answers to those two questions will save lives... yours *and* mine," he answered gravely.

"I remind you that in his book *Atkin's Nutritional Breakthrough,* Dr. Robert C. Atkin writes:

'The matchup of what we know about our immune system with what we know about cancer holds out the hope of providing the answers we have all been seeking. The question raised is a tantalizing one: If the body's immune system controls cancer, then is it not possible that the true breakthrough against cancer may be found in strengthening our immunity factors?'"

"Yes, I remember, Larry. We already have that quote in the book. Did you forget?"

"No. I just thought it was important to emphasize the point, Carter. You go along now. I see in your memory banks that you have tickets for a football game. We'll talk more later."

Bibliography

Atkins, MD, RZ: Dr. Atkins' Nutrition Breakthrough. New York: William Morrow and Co, 1981.

Gerson, M: A Cancer Therapy - Results of Fifty Cases. Delmar, CA: Totality Books, 1977.

Guyton, AC: Text Book of Medical Physiology. Philadelphia: WB Saunders Co, 1986.

Smedley, H, Sikora, K and Stepney, R: Cancer, What It Is and How It's Treated. Oxford, Great Britain: Basil Blackwell Ltd, 1985.

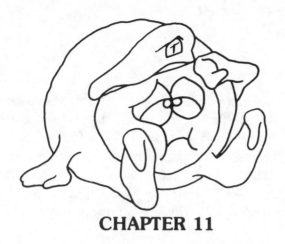

CHAPTER 11

AN IMPORTANT LESSON
FROM LARRY

"Don't eat that."

It was half-time at the Seattle Seahawks versus the Denver Broncos football game. I was doing what all redblooded football enthusiasts do at half-time, feeding my face. I was just about to enjoy a bite of the hot dog I had bought at the concession stand in the Kingdome when I heard Larry's familiar voice buzzing in my left ear.

"Where are you, Larry?" I sent the thought to him.

"I'm located in the primary visual cortex of your brain so that I can watch the game, Carter."

"What? You can see?" I was astonished.

"As long as I stay in your visual cortex, whatever you see, I see," he explained. "It's sort of like watching television. And it's a good thing for all of us that I was on guard so I can warn you not to eat that stuff."

"This hot dog?" I exclaimed in surprise. "There's nothing wrong with this hot dog, Larry. It's good food, and I'm hungry. Besides, before you get it, I have to eat it."

"I'm speaking for all the cells of your body, Carter. We don't want it."

"Why?"

"Because we can't use it. It makes a tremendous amount of work for us. We have to try to get rid of it, you see."

"That's what you have to do with all the food I eat," I said reasonably. "You have to figure out how to use it, or lose it."

"I'm not talking about the *food* you eat, Carter. I'm concerned about the junk in that hot dog that isn't food."

"Larry," I said patiently. "This is a *hot dog*, America's favorite meat product... "

"They may try to tell you that hot dogs are meat, but that one you almost bit into contains very little meat. It's made up largely of spices and awful additives, including sodium nitrate, sodium ascorbate, glucona delta lactos, and a bunch of fillers."

"Well, I know hot dogs may have a few fillers, but... "

"A few!" he exclaimed in disgust. "The fatty parts of the animal, which you normally avoid, are the only so-called 'meat' in that hot dog, Carter."

"Wait just a doggone minute, Larry. Each hot dog has to have a certain amount of protein in order to meet USDA standards."

"But to increase the protein content of that hot dog, dried milk and soy flour were added. You can bet other fillers include cereal or starchy vegetable flour."

"Larry, if you're still in my visual cortex, just look at this hot dog. It looks good, smells great, and I bet it tastes just like a hot dog is supposed to taste."

"Carter, the mustard you put on that hot dog probably contains even more chemicals and additives than the hot dog. And the bun is no better."

"What's wrong with additives?" I said in exasperation. "They make food better."

"It would be nice if you were right. But, no matter what the food industry people try to tell you, that's just not so."

"Are you telling me that food additives are dangerous to my

health?"

"No. Not all additives are dangerous just because they're added to your food. In fact, if we cells can break down an additive into healthy, useful nutrients, then we handle it just as we do any good food. But if the cells are harmed in any way, or the additive is identified by your immune defense forces as a foreign substance, it reduces our efficiency measurably. You wouldn't believe all the time and trouble we have to go to just to get rid of some of that gunk you eat. It's very important for you to remember, Carter, that anything which reduces the efficiency of your immune system increases the probability that you'll develop cancer."

"Whoa! Wait a minute here, Larry. I don't know of any scientist who would go out on a limb and say that eating hot dogs causes cancer."

"You're right. But your human scientists haven't found the answer to cancer, remember? And they're still producing more than 6,000 chemicals every year, some of which will end up as food additives."

"You're over-reacting, little buddy. The FDA has to approve a substance before they can put it in food. Surely not all of the chemicals added to our foods are dangerous, Larry."

"Don't be too sure about that. The cumulative effects of these chemicals are unknown. And the possible interaction of *combinations* of additives haven't even been considered by human scientists, Carter."

"I guess you're right, Larry. When new chemicals are investigated, they are given to lab animals one at a time in order to secure the necessary scientific data."

"More than 4,000 food additives are currently in use, Carter."

"Wow! How do you know that?"

"Because it's my responsibility to identify them when your immune defense forces encounter them in your body for the first time, Carter. Very few of these additives have any nutritional value at all. Many are simply unnecessary. What

I want to know, Carter, is this: Who is responsible for putting them in your food?"

"Additives are put in at the discretion of the food processors."

"Why do they use additives at all?"

"Well, to make their products more attractive, I guess. To keep foods fresher longer, to keep them from spoiling, to extend shelf life."

"Uh huh. Sure," he said scornfully. "I think what you're telling me, Carter, is that your food industry humans are more interested in profits than they are in pure foods."

"That's a little harsh, Larry."

"Not really. Consider this, Carter: If the only responsibility your immune system had to worry about was to search out and destroy mutant cells, cancer would not exist."

"You're going off on a tangent here, Larry. Stop changing the subject."

"I'm not changing the subject at all, Carter. I'm making a very important point. If all we had to do was keep your body clear of mutant cells, cancer would no longer exist."

"That's another very bold statement, Larry. How are you going to back this one up?"

"The immune system defense forces are intricately organized. We handle all emergencies with the expertise of supreme military strategists, but cancer is unorganized, grows slowly and erratically. All the cells of your body live in basically the same environment. Water. An ocean... no. Let's compare it to an aquarium. We live in a complex controlled environment."

"Who controls the environment?"

"You guessed it, Carter. Your cells. We obey literally thousands of rules and regulations known as feedback controls, well understood by us cells. By obeying our programming, we keep the temperature of your body at approximately 98.6 degrees, your pH balance just right, your electrical balance within acceptable ranges, and we even control the amount of water surrounding all cells."

"It sounds like a cell utopia to me," I answered.

"That's our objective, of course. But our world exists within your world. You see, the perfect cell environment would contain no pollutants. Without pollutants, your defense forces wouldn't have to work so hard to maintain homeostasis. Although there will always be mutant cells, cancer couldn't develop into a threat."

"But, unfortunately, we humans don't live in a perfect environment, so neither do our cells." I was catching on.

"You are so right, Carter. In fact, it sometimes seems to us cells that you humans are doing everything possible to pollute our internal environment. You're making it harder and harder for your immune system to do its various jobs."

"Please explain."

"That's easy, Carter. On top of running herd on mutant cells, your immune system has the responsibility of eating dead cells and eliminating all alien particles. On average, you swallow five pounds of additives every year. Most of these additives are alien particles. We have to classify each one of them in a lymph node. Then your defense forces have to deal with each one of them and eliminate them somehow."

"But, Larry," I protested, "you've always had that job. I don't see any change in your responsibilities."

"You don't? You're not old enough to remember how things used to be, Carter. Around the turn of the century, eliminating alien particles from the internal environment really wasn't a hard task for a crack team of lymphocytes. We had been doing it for thousands of years. There were very few new alien particles to identify and defend against eighty years ago. But, during the 19th century, unscrupulous food producers concealed the alteration of foods with chemical substances. Their first objective was to maintain and enhance color, then to improve or change the flavor and texture, and, of course, to extend shelf-life. This gave rise to the public's attempt to establish a consumer protection agency."

"How do you know all this?" I asked suspiciously.

"Do you remember reading Upton Sinclair's book, *The Jungle?*"

"Yes. That was required reading when I was back in high school. But I didn't get much out of it."

"That book played a major role in securing the Pure Food & Drug Act of 1906," he informed me smugly.

"You're just full of information, aren't you?" I was a bit miffed.

"More than you think, Carter. In 1958, the U.S. government authorized a food additive amendment stipulating that any substance added to a food had to be proven safe by the manufacturer before being put in foods offered for sale. Your FDA officials compiled a list of additives they called 'Generally Recognized As Safe,' or GRAS for short."

"See. The additives *are* safe."

"I wish I could agree, Carter, but that's not the case. The safety of your chemical additives is tested by using animals. But each additive is tested alone, and not in combination with other additives that might end up in the body at the same time."

"And I suppose you think that combining additives may be harmful?"

"There's no '*may be*' about it, Carter. I *know* so. Today, the average supermarket where you humans shop contains more than 8,000 items that are regarded as food."

"There's nothing wrong with variety, Larry."

"More than two-thirds of the food products in your supermarkets were never seen in a store before World War II."

"So what? We have creative scientists."

"That's my point, Carter. Don't you realize that nearly all of these newer items are processed foods products, or foods produced from a chemical formula? They are either partially or totally artificial."

"Wow! I think I'm beginning to see what you're getting at."

"Finally! I was starting to wonder. Now, why do you suppose

anybody would want to put additives into the foods you eat?"

"The purpose of additives? So that major food corporations can make more money, I suppose."

"Bingo. Food processors add preservatives to keep foods looking fresh during storage, shipping, and on the shelves of the supermarket."

"To give consumers a greater opportunity to buy their products, Larry."

"The food processors add antioxidants to inhibit the breakdown of fats and oils so they won't go rancid at room temperature."

"Less waste. Greater net profit. That's the 'American way.' "

"Antibiotics are added to extend the life of fresh foods and are also given to meat animals to make them grow more rapidly and reach market size sooner."

"Good old Yankee know-how, little buddy. Less cost for produce and meats, and a faster cash-flow."

"We're on a roll, Carter. Hormones are added to fatten up meat animals with less feed."

"That just results in more bucks-per-hoof for the slaughter house."

"You've got an answer for everything, haven't you, Carter? Those were easy, but I've got more. To develop a uniform and smooth texture, stabilizers and emulsifiers are added to creamy foods."

"Which results in consumer satisfaction; which results in repeat business and greater sales volume."

"Good. Are you aware that *sequesterants* are also found in your foods?"

"What are sequesterants?"

"They are chemicals added to separate out trace elements which might otherwise interfere with processing."

"Hmmm... Let's see. To cut factory overhead costs, which increases productivity and profitability."

"And don't forget the buffers and neutralizers, which are

added to control the acid content."

"Well, Larry, I guess the food industry is so competitive that the big boys who can afford to pay creative scientists to develop cheaper substitute foods are constantly trying to beat out the rest of the processors and get to market first with a cheaper product."

"Okay, Carter. There's more. It might surprise you to learn that the processors also use solvents to keep the other additives properly distributed; coating agents to make foods like chocolates and oranges shine; and propellants added to carbonated beverages, or to make it possible for foods with creamy textures to eject from aerosol cans."

"Lay off, Larry. I get the picture."

"I'm not through yet. The list goes on, including bleaches, moisteners, drying agents, extenders, thickeners, conditioners, curing agents, fortifiers, sweeteners, and on and on and on. Carter, you humans are supposed to possess advanced intelligence. Why do your food processors choose to poison the entire race?"

"First of all, Larry, I don't believe they know what they're doing. Second, I guess most of the time synthetic or artificial food products cost less to produce than the real thing. Synthetic food products have to cost the consumer less in order to compete in the marketplace with the real thing.

"We are children of a 'plastic' world. Imitation lime juice and lemon juice are packaged to look like plastic fruit. *Tang* is a synthetic orange juice and contains no vital trace elements. Many so-called 'fruit' punches are highly synthetic and made up of mostly artificial flavors and colors."

"Speaking of artificial colors, Carter, are you aware that *every year four million pounds* of certified dyes are added to foods manufactured in the United States?"

"No. I never thought much about it. But artificial colors aren't dangerous. Or are they?"

"In 1919, your scientists said that 'butter-yellow' was found to produce cancer in the liver. It was taken off the market."

"Gotcha, Larry! Aren't you the guy who told me that nothing 'causes' cancer."

"You're right. But your scientists don't know that. When butter-yellow is introduced into the internal environment of the cells, I'm talking about the body, it keeps the immune system forces so busy cleaning it up that the leukocytes can't get on with their regular work of chasing down mutant cells, and therefore cancer of the liver develops."

"That must have been serious."

"I'm just starting. In 1960, the certified colors FD & C Orange, and numbers 1 and 2 Red were banned because they were found to damage internal organs. And they discovered that several more of the yellow dyes caused intestinal lesions and damaged the heart."

"You're scaring me, Larry. This is almost as bad as the stuff I found out about chemotherapy drugs."

"I have some small comfort for you, Carter. Red dye #4 is restricted to use in maraschino cherries only."

"Why is that?"

"Back in 1965, they were about to ban Red dye #4 entirely. But the maraschino cherry people convinced the FDA that humans eat only one or two maraschino cherries at a time, meaning that an individual wouldn't ingest sufficient Red #4 to cause harm. You see, the scientists had determined that Red #4 harmed the adrenal glands and urinary bladders of dogs."

"Dogs! What does it do to humans?"

"I say that any damage that can be avoided is too much damage," he said forcefully. "To initiate the cancer process, remember that all a substance has to do is cause just one cell to mutate. Incidentally, maraschino cherries are flavored with synthetic maraschino, not the true maraschino liqueur which is made from the little wild cherries called marascas.

"To continue, did you know that Red dye #2 was banned entirely in the Soviet Union because it caused birth defects, impaired reproductive capabilities, and induced cancer in laboratory animals?"

"No, I didn't know that," I said thoughtfully.

"Carter, you humans have been consuming this dye in soft drinks, candies, ice cream, baked goods, cherries, and even sausages for many years. Russian experts say that only two of the certified dyes used in the U.S. are harmless."

"All right, Larry. I give up. You've made your point. Everything we eat is somehow harmful to our health."

"Not everything, Carter. Just 'people' food. That's what I call the good food that processors have altered. But there's still plenty of good 'cell-food' available, if you know where to find it."

"Cell-food! This time you've gone too far, Larry. I suppose next you're going to tell me to get my groceries in a cell-food supermarket where all you little cells do your shopping."

"What a good idea, Carter!" he enthused. "I'd certainly patronize such a store, if it were possible. I only wish we cells *could* do our own shopping, instead of having to depend on you humans for the nutrients we need."

"Well, forget it, Larry," I said witheringly. "I wouldn't shop at a cell-food store, even if one existed."

"You don't have to, Carter. There's plenty of cell-food at your supermarket. You just have to know what to bring home... and what to avoid."

I suddenly remembered the uneaten paper-wrapped bundle still clutched in my hand. "Hey! It's all your fault, Larry! After talking all this time, my hot dog got cold."

"Good! Throw it away. You don't need it, and I surely don't want it."

"But I'm hungry. The nerve cells of my stomach are telling me so."

"Buy popcorn," he advised promptly. "That's cell-food. But don't let them put any of that disgusting synthetic yellow gunk on it they call 'butter-flavored oil.' And hurry up, Carter, or we'll miss the second half of the game. For some reason I can't fathom, you seem to get a kick out of seeing humans crashing into other humans."

"Don't be sarcastic, Larry. Football is a great game." I glanced at my watch and dashed for the popcorn vendor. "I've got a great idea, Larry," I said as I hurried back to my seat. "On the way home, we'll stop at the supermarket and you can show me what cell-food looks like."

"You're learning, Carter," he answered approvingly.

Bibliography

Atkins, MD, RZ: Dr. Atkins' Nutrition Breakthrough. New York: William Morrow and Co, 1981.

Fischer, WL: How to Fight Cancer and Win. Canfield, Ohio: Fischer Publishing Corporation, 1987.

Guyton, AC: Text Book of Medical Physiology. Philadelphia: WB Saunders Co, 1986.

Robinson, CH: Fundamentals in Normal Nutrition. New York: MacMillian, 1973.

Svacha, AJ, Wesson, NC and Waslein, CI: Effect of Egg Intake and Tobacco Smoking on Serum Cholesterol. Fed Proc 33:690, 1974.

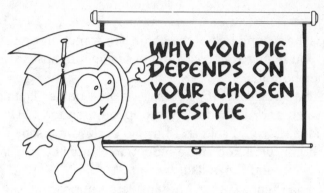

WHY YOU DIE
DEPENDS ON
YOUR CHOSEN
LIFESTYLE

CHAPTER 12

SHOPPING WITH LARRY

"Okay, Larry, tell me what you thought of the football game."

"Ridiculous. A total waste of good energy, Carter."

I wasn't about to let him spoil my good mood. "Wait a minute, Larry. We won!"

" '*We*' won? I wasn't aware that *we* were playing, Carter."

"Our team won... the team we were cheering for, Larry."

"You mean the team *you* were cheering for, Carter. I just don't understand humans, I guess. You and thousands of other humans go to a stadium to watch other humans try to destroy each other's bodies while you eat things which destroy *your* bodies. And now you say you *'won?'* Think for a minute about all the repair work millions of cells will have to do during the next few days just to fix up the humans on both sides."

"Oh, Larry," I said with a sigh. My good mood was fading fast. "It's only a game."

"And that's how you humans look at life, isn't it, Carter. You 'play' until the end, and then that's it. Who wins then? My entire life is dedicated to keeping you alive. And I'm not getting much help from you either," he said heatedly.

"I can't believe this," I said. "Here I am sitting in my own car in the parking lot of my neighborhood supermarket arguing with 'myself' about the meaning of the game of life. Look Larry, nobody gets out of this life alive."

"You're right, Carter. The only real choice you have is how and when you die."

"Are you telling me I have a choice?" I asked incredulously, my annoyance forgotten.

"Most of the time, yes."

"Now that's going to take some explanation."

"Not much. If you decided to die today, you could easily drive head on into the path of an oncoming truck."

"Oh, get serious, Larry."

"No, Carter. *You* get serious. Most of the time the way you die depends on your chosen lifestyle and the knowledge you have about the way your body functions."

"People die of many causes," I protested.

"Most of which are controllable, Carter," he said flatly, "including dying of cancer."

"Okay, Larry. I'm ready to listen to what's bugging a bug." I smiled at my quip.

"I'm not a 'bug,' and you're not funny. That's a perfect example of what I mean. Here we are in the middle of writing a book about what could be the most important medical breakthrough of any century, and you still won't take me seriously."

"Wrong, Larry. I do take you seriously. It's just that I get kind of embarrassed when people catch me talking to myself. They must think I'm out of my mind."

"Out of your mind and into your body. What's wrong with that?" he shot back.

"Nothing. It's just that some people don't understand."

"You can say that again! In fact, nobody understands. That's why we're writing this book."

"You're right, Larry. I keep forgetting that our best scientists have only known about the DNA for 25 years, and the relationship between the DNA and cancer for less than 10 years. You cells have been coping with cancer very ably and have had it under control for thousands of years."

"Very good, Carter. There's hope for you yet. What have you learned so far?"

"You want me to tell you *now*? Sitting here in the parking lot getting funny looks from everyone that passes by? Give me a break, Larry."

"Just a summary, if you please. *Professor* Carter."

"Yes, well... here goes: Cancer has been misdiagnosed as a family of diseases, but it's not a disease at all."

"Good," he approved. "What is it?"

"Cancer is a symptom of an inefficient immune system."

"Right. And why is the true knowledge of cancer so important?"

"We won't have to spend vast amounts of time and money on obsolete cancer therapies that have been proven more destructive than cancer itself."

"Excellent. Go on."

"Nothing causes cancer. Any chemical classified scientifically as carcinogenic or mutagenic can only cause certain cells to mutate."

"Why is that important?"

"We won't have to fear any chemicals classified as carcinogenic."

"Why is that?"

"Because in order for a cell to qualify as a cancer cell, it has to mutate twice. In the meantime, mutant cells are being hunted down ceaselessly by a very efficient army of millions of lymphocytes."

"What else?"

"The healthy immune system is well equipped to control all mutant cells and all foreign invaders, plus handling the normal cleanup of dead and dying cells."

"The bottom line now, Carter. What is the answer to cancer?"

"What?" I screeched. "Larry, that's what this book is all about. Aren't you supposed to tell us?"

"Nobody will believe a cell, Carter. It has to come from a human."

"They won't believe me either," I said dejectedly.

"They don't have to. This book is so well documented that all they have to do is research the sources listed in the bibliography. I ask you again. What is the answer to cancer?"

"A healthy, active immune system."

"That wasn't so hard, was it?"

"I guess not. But there's so much more to learn." I had a sudden disquieting thought. "You're not going to leave us, are you, Larry?"

"Not if you don't want me to, Carter."

"I don't," I answered quickly. "I still need to know what I can do to help make my immune defense forces more efficient. That's the *real* bottom line, isn't it Larry?"

"Of course. I thought you'd never figure it out, Carter. First, we start with cell-food. All cells need cell-food. Let's go into the store and see what we can find."

"Okay, Larry. We're in. Show me where the best cell-food is."

"You're in the wrong place, Carter."

"Well, we had to start somewhere. This is the center of the store. Direct me."

"I don't see anything nutritious around here, Carter. All I see are cardboard boxes, cans, and bottles of stuff."

"This can right here has peaches in it. You have to read the labels, silly."

"You read labels. I don't. The producers want you to believe what they put on their labels. How did those peaches get in there?"

"After the peaches were picked, I guess they were shipped to a cannery somewhere and put in the can."

"And what temperature do you suppose those peaches were subjected to before they were sealed up in that tin can?"

"I don't know. Around 200 degrees Fahrenheit, I imagine. Why? What difference does it make?"

"Ahh, Carter. You *are* woefully lacking in important knowledge. Some very vital enzymes that I need are destroyed at temperatures over 120 degrees. Those peaches cannot be considered decent cell-food. Let's go for the real thing."

"Where?"

"Carter, the perimeter of most stores is where you usually find cell-food."

"I see." I said thoughtfully. "What you're telling me is that fresh fruits and vegetables are good cell-foods."

"Of course, Carter," he answered patiently. "Who made them?"

"The cells of the plants."

"Very good," he approved. "Do the cells of the plants know how to produce fruit and vegetables after their own kind?"

"Yes." He was leading me by the nose.

"Do cells of plants include all of the vitamins, minerals, enzymes, and proteins necessary to produce fruits, grains, and vegetables?"

"That's obvious, Larry."

"Because fresh foods are the end result of the best that any plant can offer, they are complete cell-foods and contain all the 75-plus basic nutrients your cells need to keep your body healthy, Carter."

"Terrific!" I enthused. "Are you telling me that the fruit or vegetable produced by a single plant has *all* the nutrients you cells need to keep me healthy?"

"No. But a combination of fresh fruits and vegetables does."

"But what about protein? Don't I have to eat meat or meat byproducts to get you the complete protein we both need?"

"Tell me this, Carter: Why do your cells need protein?"

"For energy, I suppose."

"Oh, yes," he said witheringly. "That *is* what you humans have been taught, isn't it? Cells do need protein, because all proteins are made up of the 22 amino acids that are required by your cells so we can manufacture your own protein. All the protein you need for the hairs on your head, your fingernails, bones, muscles, skin tissue, and even mucous membranes is manufactured by us cells."

"We have been taught that proteins are the building-blocks of the cells," I said defensively.

"No. The 22 *amino acids* are the building-blocks of the cells. Proteins are the source of amino acids. All cells, plant or animal, have cell membranes composed of proteins and lipids, or fats. All cells have a nucleus and DNA, which is made up of nucleo-protein. All organelles, the structures inside the cells, are composed of protein. You don't have to look far to find protein, Carter. It's in everything natural and unprocessed that you eat. Now, name me some more good cell-foods."

"Nuts and grains, I suppose."

"Excellent, Carter! This is going to be easier than I thought. Why did you name nuts and grains?"

"Because they are the very essence of the plant. The grain is one of the primary reasons for its existence.."

"You're beginning to get the picture, Carter. Congratulations! Plant a grain of wheat, add water and sunlight, and the cells of that kernel of wheat know exactly how to produce a new plant, including the roots, stock, leaves, and ear."

"Is wheat a complete cell-food then?" I asked.

"For the wheat plant, yes. But humans are not plants. Wheat doesn't have *all* the amino acids we cells need to manufacture human protein. But when you eat wheat in combination with other types of plants, the combination becomes complete cell-food. Carter, please walk around the perimeter of this store and let's check out what they're offering in the way of cell-food today."

"Right. There's the fruits and nuts. Here are all the fresh vegetables. What about fish?"

"Excellent."

"How about chicken and turkey?"

"Both are good cell-foods, provided they aren't polluted with antibiotics, growth hormones, insecticides and pesticides, or contaminated with fecal bacteria and worse in the processing."

"Oh, yes. I remember seeing a program on 60 Minutes showing how chickens are processed. It was disgusting to find out that USDA regulations are being flaunted and to learn that there's a possibility that the chicken we find in the supermarket might be dangerous to our health."

"There's an easy answer to that dilemma, Carter. Just find a kosher butcher."

"I'm not Jewish, Larry. But I have heard that processors of kosher foods have to 'answer to a higher authority.' "

"We cells don't care how or where you humans worship, Carter. But we do want clean uncontaminated nutrition," he said pointedly.

"There really is a difference in the processing then?" I asked.

"Absolutely. Standard chicken processing calls for all the slaughtered chickens to be dumped in a vat of scalding hot water, heads, feathers, claws, and all, as the first step. These are dirty birds, Carter. A chicken house is full of chicken feces and worse. The feathers and feet of the slaughtered birds are filthy and contaminated. The function of this first 'bath' is to wash off all the outer pollutants, but the stagnant water itself is quickly contaminated and grows more and more polluted as more and more batches of birds go through it. Then, too, the hotter the water is, the greasier it gets as surface fats and oil are leached out."

I shuddered at the mental picture he was painting for me. "Ugh," I said as I made a face. "Kosher processing is different, I hope."

"Oh my, yes. Kosher processors use a fresh bath of ice water for each batch of birds. That's good in itself, but the very best kosher processors use a forceful spray of fresh tap water to wash away all the outer contamination on the birds. All those clinging globs of feces and filth are washed away and down the drain. Kosher chickens aren't permitted to slosh around in a polluted bath of scalding hot contaminated water."

"That does sound a lot more appetizing," I acknowledged. "Are there other differences too?"

"Sure. After picking and gutting, standard processors dump the birds into another vat of stagnant water before they go into large chillers to cool them down quickly. The problem with these large refrigerators is that the birds are packed in tightly and a lot of them get mashed up pretty badly, resulting in blood bruises and the like. And the birds in the center of the mass take a long time to cool down, giving bacteria time to grow. On the other hand, kosher processing calls for the birds to be put into aging vats... "

"Aging vats? You mean kosher chickens are 'old,' Larry?" I interrupted.

"No, of course not, Carter. The aging vats are filled with what is known as 'slush,' a circulating mixture of ice and water. Instead of being thrown into a chiller, kosher chickens go into the slush and are cooled quickly and uniformly.

"But the most important difference in kosher processing is the final step. Because Jewish people are forbidden by religious law to ingest what is known as 'lifeline blood,' kosher chickens are handled in a very special way. The internal cavities are filled with coarse kosher salt, and the birds are packed in additional kosher salt... and held that way for at least an hour."

"That's interesting, Larry. But what's the reason behind it?"

"The Torah teaches that this salting-down draws off all fresh 'lifeline' blood and renders the meat suitable for eating. This method of handling meat was prescribed by Jewish law about 4,000 years ago, Carter. And there's another healthful benefit to be gained as well."

"What's that?"

"What's the oldest natural remedy for a sore throat, Carter?"

"Aren't you getting a little off the track here, Larry?"

"Not at all. Just answer the question."

"Let's see. My grandmother always said gargling with warm salt water was the best way to heal a sore throat."

"She was right. And the last time you had a tooth pulled, didn't I hear your dentist tell you to rinse with warm salt water? Salt is one of the oldest germ fighters around. It kills bacteria. That's why kosher chickens have triple the shelf-life of chickens processed the usual way. Ordinary fresh chickens last about three or four days, but fresh kosher chickens are shelf-safe for up to three weeks. Of course, no matter how the birds are processed, both have to be kept well refrigerated."

"You've convinced me, Larry. The next time my wife sends me out to buy chicken, I'll shop 'kosher.' Thanks for the tip. But to get back on the subject of cell-food, is it safe to say that just about everything that's fresh and natural is good cell-food?"

"That's a pretty good generalization, Carter."

"Except for eggs, right? Eggs are too high in cholesterol."

"That's just more human propaganda," he said scornfully. "Sales hype. Cholesterol scare tactics. Carter, eggs are some of the best high-protein cell-food around. If you leave a fertilized egg in the nest for 27 days, what do you get?"

"A chicken."

"Of course. Complete with eyes, beak, brain, muscles, skin, feathers, bones, gizzard, and everything else. The smart little cells of the egg produce all the cells that are needed to make up a living chicken without any outside help."

"But what about the cholesterol?"

"Oh, Carter," he sighed. "You humans are so dense sometimes. You *need* cholesterol to digest some of the foods you eat. All of us cells require a measure of cholesterol. If you don't eat it, we just manufacture what we need in quantities of up to one-and-a-half grams per day. We manufacture 95 percent of the cholesterol in your body anyway."

"But if I eat too many eggs, won't the cholesterol levels in my blood increase dangerously, turn into atherosclerotic plaque, and clog up my veins?"

"Certainly not. The yolk of the egg contains the highest concentration of *lecithin* found in nature."

"What's lecithin?" I asked.

"Lecithin is one of the natural fats, a lipid, that helps keep cholesterol in suspension. As long as you're eating the good cell-foods we need to process cholesterol efficiently, you don't have to be concerned about the cholesterol levels in your blood."

"And what might those cell-foods be, oh mighty mite?"

"The foods that contain the essential fatty acids are *very* important to us cells, Carter. Your scientists have dubbed the essential fatty acids *linoleic* acid and *linolenic* acid. And 'essential' means just that. The cells of your body cannot manufacture linoleic or linolenic acid from any other nutrients. We have to depend on you to deliver them to us. And when you don't, you're creating all kinds of health problems that we can't deal with very effectively. We need the essential fatty acids every day."

I could feel that he was deadly serious. "What do these essential fatty acids do for me, Larry?"

"Many good things, Carter. Because we're talking about how your body manages cholesterol, let's explore that function first. The melting point of cholesterol is 300 degrees F. At your normal body temperature of 98.6 degrees, cholesterol travels through the bloodstream sluggishly and sticky bits catch on arterial walls, eventually building into atherosclerotic plaque and clogging the passageways. But in the presence of the essential fatty acids, cholesterol is liquified at temperatures well below your normal body temperature. In its liquid form, cholesterol travels easily through the bloodsteam and cannot develop into harmful atherosclerotic plaque.

"But the essential fatty acids do a lot more than that. All around the world, scientists are busy in their laboratories investigating the benefits of the essentials. British researchers have found that sheep given linseed oil with a grossly high-fat diet didn't exhibit the harmful substances which develop when fats can't be processed by the body. Because it's the richest source known of linoleic and linolenic acids, most scientists are using linseed oil to discover why the body needs the essential fatty acids.

"In Poland, scientists have reported that replacing saturated fats in the diet with the essentials offers strong protection against heart disease. And in Patna, India, experiments with rabbits showed that animals given linseed oil were free of high cholesterol levels and atherosclerotic plaque. The Indian scientists reached the conclusion that the properties of linseed oil were superior to other polyunsaturated fats. Australian researchers have shown that the essential fatty acids protect against high blood pressure.

"However, since this book is about cancer, I think what's really important for you to understand is why we cells need the essential fatty acids in our fight against mutant cells. In Austria, Poland, and Germany, human scientists are showing what we've known all along. The active properties in linseed oil work against mutant and malignant cells without harming my extended family, the white blood cells of the immune defense forces.

"When cancer gets a toehold in the body, Carter, the cells of the blood undergo unhealthy changes. The blood of seriously ill people, including cancer patients, is always deficient in linoleic acid and the phosphatides needed for normal cell division, and is lacking in albumin, a blood-producing lipoprotein. Albumin is a mating of linoleic acid and sulphur-based proteins. Without this vital combination of the essential fatty acids and sulphurated proteins, the blood shows an unhealthy, greenish substance in place of the red oxygen-carrying hemoglobin. Without hemoglobin, the cells of the entire body become starved for oxygen.

"A German biochemist by the name of Dr. Johanna Budwig

has been treating cancer patients for over ten years with a combination of crude linseed oil and cottage cheese. The linseed oil provides the essential fatty acids, and the cottage cheese provides sulphur-based proteins. Dr. Budwig has been using this combination for a decade in clinical application in her private practice with great success. By closely monitoring blood samples of her patients, Dr. Budwig has proven that supplying the body with crude linseed oil combined with cottage cheese results in some miraculous changes in the constituents of the blood. This dietary supplement gradually replaces the vital phosphatides and albumin missing in the blood, and the greenish alien elements give way to healthy red blood cells.

"All this scientific research is very gratifying, Carter. It's nice to know that you humans are getting on the right track at last. But it's even more important to you and me and the trillions of cells that make up your body to make sure that your diet includes the essential fatty acids right now, *before* things go haywire. You give us the ammunition we need, and we cells can nip mutant cells in the bud and *keep* you healthy."

"That's pretty impressive documentation, Larry. I'm convinced. Point me to the shelf where the essential fatty acids are and I'll take some home today."

"Aye, there's the rub, Carter. It's not so easy to put linoleic and linolenic acid on the menu when you're shopping in an ordinary supermarket. In order of their importance, the essential fatty acids are found in raw linseeds, pumpkin seeds, soybeans, and walnuts."

"I think you might be wrong, little buddy. If the essential fatty acids are *fats*, there's no problem shopping in the supermarket. Every supermarket in the nation is well stocked with a great variety of all kinds of margarines and vegetable oils. At least some margarines are made with soy oil, if not linseed, pumpkin, or walnut oils, and I bet I can find a bottle of soy oil on the shelf somewhere. No big deal."

"Oh, but it is a big deal, Carter. The way you humans produce artificial dietary fats is frightening to me. The end result is a conglomeration of alien particles that I have to get rid of somehow. And, believe me, it's not easy."

"I don't understand, Larry."

"Okay, let's take hydrogenated and partially hydrogenated fats. Your food processors put that poison in just about everything,"

"Poison! Nonsense, Larry. The entire civilized world has been eating margarine and using vegetable oils for years. There can't be anything wrong with them"

"Oh, but there is, Carter," he answered grimly. "In order to produce vegetable oil, the artificial fats industry starts with some perfectly natural seeds. By the time they have been cooked and subjected to high-friction grinding and a chemical-extraction process and bottled in the U.S. as 'cold-pressed' and 'unrefined' oils, very few of the good nutrients remain, traces of chemicals are left behind, and all the enzymes that the cells of your body need have been destroyed.

"As if that's not bad enough," he continued forcefully, "the hydrogenation process where all the molecules of the oil are saturated with hydrogen in the presence of a metal catalyst at excessively high temperature renders the final product completely useless as far as nutrition goes. But the *partial* hydrogenation process is even worse. In order to harden a liquid fat and produce margarine or solid shortening, the hydrogenation process is halted when the mass begins to solidify. This leaves behind all sorts of erratically hydrogenated molecules which are totally alien to the body.

"These chemically-altered fats are garbage and do not provide the essential fatty acids. They add up to yet more enemies that the immune forces have to defend against when we *should* be cleaning up mutant cells, Carter. And you humans wonder why cancer is on the rise!"

"You're scaring me, Larry. Stop hollering. If linseed oil is such good preventive medicine and gives you guys the essential fatty acids my body needs, point me to it!"

"I can't 'point you to it,' Carter. We're in the wrong store. You have to find a health food store that offers raw, unrefined cold-pressed virgin linseed oil. Unfortunately, *only* the cold-pressed variety is correctly processed and handled and still retains its full complement of beneficial fatty acids. I hate to hammer home my point, but the cold-pressed so-called unrefined oils produced by most American manufacturers just don't measure up. The virgin linseed oil you want is *C-Leinosan Linseed Oil.* Leinosan is an all-organic oil. It is carefully cold-pressed, and contains a rich supply of both linoleic and linolenic acids, the essential fatty acids that benefit your body."

"Okay, Larry. I hear and obey. I've made a mental note to find C-Leinosan Brand linseed oil. I promise you that I'll throw out everything in the house that's made with hydrogenated or partially hydrogenated fats. But let's continue. What about sugar? Is sugar good cell-food, Larry?"

"You bet it is. In fact, everything we cells use to create energy has to be converted into blood sugar, or *glucose,* before we can use it properly."

"Then what you're saying is that sugar is good for my body."

"Your body can't function without it, Carter. But there are several kinds of sugar. *Fructose* and *dextrose* are both found in fruits and honey; *lactose* is milk-sugar; and *sucrose* is the type of sugar you get from maple sap, sugar cane, and beets."

"Then what's wrong with eating sugar?"

"In its natural state, there's nothing wrong with sugar because nature combines it with vitamins, minerals, an assortment of enzymes, and important activators and nutritive factors. But when sugar is refined into those white crystals you put in your sugar bowl, it's 99 percent pure carbon with a bit of hydrogen and oxygen. Every last trace of the vitamins and minerals and other nutrients have been removed.

"Because refined sugar is so concentrated, it floods into your internal environment unchecked. Sugar drastically upsets homeostasis and makes it extremely hard for the cells of your body to do what they're supposed to do. In order to function properly, we have to quickly stabilize your blood sugar levels. Eating refined carbohydrate foods loaded with concentrated sugar puts an unbearable strain on the cells of the pancreas and the liver, and it sometimes pushes those vital organs beyond their physical capabilities."

I couldn't wait to get home and share all this exciting news with my wife, Bonnie. I came in laden with fresh whole foods. While I passed on all that Larry had taught me, Bonnie and I went ruthlessly through the cupboards, refrigerator, and freezer and pitched out at least a hundred dollars worth of commercially-processed food products that Larry persisted in calling 'poison.' Our kitchen was now well stocked with nature's bounty.

"Cell-food really isn't so hard to find when you know where to look for it," I mused aloud.

Larry's ready answer buzzed in my right ear. "You're right, Carter. Even your scientists are beginning to recognize the concept. Walter S. Ross, editor of *Cancer News*, which is, as you know, an American Cancer Society publication, says that since the 1960s, scientists have been investigating food groups and the whole spectrum of nutrients, vitamins, minerals, and even food additives in the hope of pinpointing cancer-causing factors. More recently, studies have also focused on the protective effects certain food substances may have against the cancer process. The main emphasis of the research is on natural cancer-inhibitors, including beta-carotene, vitamins A, C, and E, and the trace mineral, selenium."

"That's good to know, Larry. Soon they'll be able to tell us what vitamin supplements we should buy and in what amounts we need to take them"

"Oh, pooh, Carter. We cells already know more than your

human scientists do about what you need to keep your immune system army healthy. And you must be very, very careful when you select dietary supplements," he cautioned. "A lot of them, even some you find in health food stores, are chemicalized and full of preservatives, sugars, starches, fillers, and artificial colors and flavors. We'll talk about some of the good supplements a little later, but right now I want to 'play mother' and coax you to eat your vegetables.

"Carter, according to dietary studies made in different parts of the world, the incidence of breast, colon, and prostate cancer is significantly lower among people who eat lots of fiber-rich vegetables. Even the American Cancer Society says that fiber is a natural cancer preventive. Walter Troll, Professor of Environmental Medicine at New York University, suggests that vegetables contain certain substances capable of inhibiting cancer in man."

"That's exciting news, Larry. What are these substances?"

"Cell-foods, of course, although the professor doesn't call them by that name. It doesn't surprise me to hear that your human scientists have found that seed vegetables, the vegetables whose edible parts are the seeds or tubers, contain compounds that seem to intercept the activity of tumor promoters."

"How about giving me some examples," I answered thoughtfully.

"Sure. That's easy. Dried beans, chickpeas, cereal grains, and potatoes are good examples of what I'm talking about, Carter. Your researchers have found that when rats bred to be susceptible to breast cancer are fed soybeans, the onset of breast cancer is greatly reduced."

"This is excellent information, Larry. Thank you."

"Hey, don't mention it, Carter. If you practice what I preach, it will make my life a lot easier."

"Right. From now on, I'm going to eat only fruits and vegetables."

"I don't believe you're hearing me, Carter. It won't do either one of us any good if you adopt some 'fad' diet."

"What do you mean?" I asked anxiously. "I thought you said... "

"You haven't been paying attention, Carter," he interrupted. "Let me give you an example. For instance, natural vitamin A is present in animal foods, including whole milk, liver, and egg yolks. But, when you don't take in enough animal nutrition, your smart little cells know how to produce vitamin A from beta-carotene. Beta-carotene is known to your scientists as the precursor of vitamin A."

"That sounds like it comes from carrots," I remarked.

"Right. Carrots are a good source of beta-carotene. But you also find it in other deep yellow and orange fruits and vegetables, including apricots, squash, and sweet potatoes. The dark green vegetables, such as spinach, kale, and broccoli, also offer substantial beta-carotene."

"Should I be taking vitamin A supplements?"

"I'd rather you didn't, Carter. As long as you take in vitamin A from natural sources, you'll never have to worry about overdoing it. Vitamin A is fat-soluble and we store it in the liver for you," he explained. "But we can only handle a certain amount at a time. Over a period of time, high doses of vitamin A can become toxic.

"And you need the fiber vegetables provide, too. Fiber, what your grandmother used to call 'roughage,' helps keep your colon from building up toxic matter which pollutes our internal environment by migrating through the walls of your intestinal tract."

"Do I have to eat all my vegetables raw?"

"No. But, generally speaking, the more you cook vegetables, the more nutrients and enzymes are destroyed. The cruciferous vegetables of the cabbage family, like cauliflower, broccoli, and brussels sprouts, can be eaten cooked or raw. These vegetables contain a group of compounds known as *indoles* which can survive cooking temperatures. Whether you prefer them cooked or raw, do eat them. Indole compounds help us fight several types of cancers," he said seriously.

"I get the picture, Larry. Let me see if I've got it straight. The bottom line is that whole natural foods are good cell-foods. What you want me to avoid are the overprocessed, additive-laden, chemicalized manufactured food products that you cells have a hard time dealing with."

"That's absolutely right, Carter." he approved. "If you stop shoveling in alien elements that the cells of your immune system defense forces have to spend time identifying, chasing down, and eliminating, we can concentrate on destroying mutant cells before they can develop into a life-threatening cancer colony. If you do your part, we can keep your body clean, free of cancer, and functioning at top efficiency. That's a promise."

"I really appreciate that, Larry," I answered fervently. Truer words were never spoken.

"Off to bed with you, Carter. I have rounds to make. You need rest. I have another concept I want to explain to you tomorrow and I'm sure you're going to think I'm off my rocker. It just might take all my powers of persuasion to convince you. I want your mind fresh and rested and ready."

I drifted off to sleep trying to figure out what he had up his sleeve ready to spring on me next.

Bibliography

Biesel, ND, WR: Nutrient Effects on Immunologic Functions. Journal American Medical Association, January 1981.

Burack, ND, WR: Lies and Statistics. Medical World News, August 1979.

Passwater, PhD, R: Cancer and Its Nutritional Therapies. New Canaan, Conn: Keats Pub, 1978.

Pfeiffer, CC: Mental and Elemental Nutrients. New Canaan: Keats Publishing Inc, 1975.

Svacha, AJ, Wesson, NC, and Waslein, CI: Effect of Egg Intake and Tobacco Smoking on Serum Cholesterol. Fed Proc, 33:690, 1974.

CHAPTER 13

LARRY EXPLAINS CELLULAR EXERCISE

"All right, Larry. You've got my curiosity aroused. What's this new concept you were talking about yesterday?"

"First we'll have what you teachers call a 'pop quiz.' Let's review. Tell me what you learned on your shopping excursion yesterday, Carter."

I sighed and realized why my students hated it when I popped a pop quiz on them.

"Okay, if I must, I must, *Professor* Lymphocyte. You've made me see that all the overprocessed and chemicalized foods that the peoples of the civilized countries of the world have been eating in ever-increasing varieties since the turn of the century are really full of alien substances that have been giving you guys a fit. I understand now that I've been overloading the capabilities of my immune defense forces by forcing you to defend against all these foreign particles."

"You're a quick study, Carter. That's very good. What else?"

"The 75 trillion cells that form my body need cell-food. I have to admit, Larry, eating cell-food is a simple concept that certainly makes sense. But why is it taking our scientists so long to recognize the food factor as the answer to cancer?" I asked.

"Probably because it's not the complete answer, Carter."

"There's more?"

"You bet! Another way you can assist your two-pound army of lymphocytes is by cell-exercise."

"Cell-exercise!" I was astonished. "What else do you guys want, little buddy? I suppose next you'll be asking me for a sauna, a pool, and a massage."

"A massage would be great, but we don't need the pool. We have our own."

"Oh, yes. You do have your own 'pool.' Your environment is water. Okay, cell-exercise. Let's see. I do push-ups, run-in-place, work out on my rowing machine, jog, ride my exercise bike, and rebound. But you can't do that stuff because you don't have arms or legs, right?"

"Right, Carter. I have pseudopodium instead."

"To each his own. You told me about your pseudo-whatever awhile back, but I guess I need a refresher course."

"The pseudopodium is our answer to your arms and legs," he answered readily. "I can project my pseudopodium far out, away from my cell body, and then follow it. Many times, I attach it to some surrounding tissue. Then, when my ectoplasm contracts, I literally pull myself along."

"How many pseudopodi do you have?" I asked curiously, trying to form a mental picture as we talked.

"As many as I need. I can extend one or more in any direction, but usually in response to a chemical or physical stimulus, an influx of positive chemical ions caused by dead or dying cells, for instance. In the case of cancer cells, the chemical signal they give off is caused by the rapid production of foreign proteins not identifiable as part of your body. And, with my pseudopodium, I can surround small, dead particles before I begin eating them."

"Okay, that's clear. But how can I provide you cells with

some exercise? You're floating in water. You don't have gravity to contend with."

"On the contrary, Carter. Every living thing on this sweet earth has to contend with gravity. It's gravity that keeps the planet earth in orbit around the sun, and the moon in orbit around the earth. Tides rise and fall with the interplay of gravity between the earth and moon."

"Sure, every schoolchild knows that, Larry. But what does gravity have to do with exercise?"

"Oh, Carter. Sometimes I wonder how you ever became a teacher." He sighed in exasperation. "How can you understand the concept of cellular exercise, when you don't understand human exercise?"

"Of course I understand human exercise, Larry. Exercise is an activity designed to make you sweat."

"Wrong. Sweating has nothing to do with exercise."

"Okay, see if you like this one better: Exercise is what we do to force our muscles to become stronger or else. If it doesn't make us hurt, it doesn't work."

"Wrong again. You don't have to hurt to be physically fit, Carter. In fact, if you hurt the next day, you did something wrong."

I tried again. "Humans exercise to tear down the weak cells of muscles to make room for stronger cells that will take their place. That's why we have been taught to exercise vigorously only three times a week. It usually takes two days for the body to recuperate," I explained helpfully.

He exploded. "That's abominable! It's wrong and extremely taxing on your immune system forces. Have you forgotten that one of the jobs of your lymphocyte army is to clean up dead cells? Destroying good cells needlessly with the wrong kind of exercise is unhealthy for your whole body. Think, man! You're talking about my extended family. Wouldn't it be more efficient, not to mention more humane, to concentrate on *strengthening* weak cells, instead of deliberately destroying them?"

"But our physical fitness experts tell us that it's important to exercise continuously for at least twenty minutes while keeping our heart pulse rate at 80 percent of its maximum capability. Otherwise, the exercise won't do our cardiovascular system any good. That's known as the 'Target Zone,' Larry. It's in *all* the exercise books. It must be right," I protested.

"Wrong. Do you believe everything you read, Carter?"

"If we can't believe the written words of our scientific experts, who can we believe?"

"I can see we're in real trouble right now."

"Okay, big mouth. If you're so smart, tell me your view of exercise. And don't tell me to do jumping jacks on my pseudopodium."

"First, let's establish once and for all that every cell in your body does need exercise and will benefit from activity."

"How do you propose to do that, Larry?"

"Your human scientists have written reams on the subject, Carter. If we go to the medical books, will that satisfy you?"

"I suppose so," I answered reluctantly, not sure where he was leading me this time.

"All right. *Gray's Anatomy,* a basic medical book, states:
'One of the characteristics of living organisms is their
ability to react to changes in their environment by
an appropriate response, which may be chemical,
electrical, photic, or mechanical.' "

"I remember reading an old *Gray's Anatomy* awhile back, Larry. But I don't think I remember reading that passage."

"It's in the 1973 British Edition, and begins on page 474."

"I'll take your word for it. Is there more?"

"Yes, the passage continues:
'All such responses involve the utilization of metabolic
energy by some sort of effector system. Several types
of effector systems exist. One, common to probably
all nucleated cells, is that which produces cytoplasmic

streaming, exemplified particularly well in unicellular organisms, such as the amoeba, the macrophages, and the lymphocytes.' "

"Okay. You just proved to me that you can move. I didn't doubt you, Larry."

"Allow me to go on, Carter. You'll find that you and I both depend on the very same molecular method for movement."

"You must be wrong this time, little buddy. I don't slide around like you do. I have legs for movement and support."

"We'll let *Gray's Anatomy* explain:
'Other examples of mechanical effectors include the muscle cells. It is interesting that in both these examples, the proteins *actin* and *myosin* are present.' "

"What are actin and myosin proteins? I've never heard of either of them."

"I was just about to tell you, Carter, but you persist in interrupting," he said tartly. "Actin and myosin are the molecules of contraction. They work together. When calcium ions and ATP energy are added, the actin molecule moves inside the myosin molecule, causing a contraction. This is how your muscles are able to contract."

"And when the actin and myosin molecules inside the muscle contract, the cells contract."

"Right. When the muscle cells contract, your muscle contracts and moves your arm or leg or whatever part you want to move."

"So muscle contraction is a function of the actin and myosin protein molecules inside the muscle cells. Is that right?"

"You got it."

"Got what?"

"The point I was trying to make, you dunderhead!"

"I did?"

"Yes. In the endoplasm, or gel, of all lymphocytes are numerous microfilaments composed of actin and myosin molecules which interact with each other to cause a contraction. The same effect occurs inside all of your muscles, Carter."

"Are you telling me now that you have muscles, Larry?" I was stunned at the thought.

"How else do you suppose we are able to move?"

"Are you going to tell me next that you need exercise to keep your muscles strong?"

"Carter, all cells need exercise. Surprisingly, we need the same kind of exercise you humans do."

"But we've already established the fact that the usual forms of exercise are out of the question for you cells. You just aren't built like a human."

"I'm not talking about the synthetic exercise that you humans have dreamed up, Carter. I'm talking about the real thing. Cellular exercise," he said emphatically.

"Cellular exercise," I mused. "I've never heard of that."

"That's probably because you're not a cell. Now listen closely: If all the cells of your body become 10 percent stronger because of a cell-exercise, what would happen to you?"

"I'd be 10 percent stronger, of course," I answered promptly.

"Then wouldn't it be a good idea for you to learn what exercise makes us cells stronger?"

"Obviously," I agreed. "But there must be a great deal of difference between cell-exercise and human exercise, Larry. There are so many different types of exercise. People use different exercises to attain different objectives."

"But there is a common denominator, Carter."

"What is it?" I asked curiously.

"All living organisms have the ability to react to changes in their environment."

"So what we do is change the cellular environment?"

"Right. Now, what's the greatest physical force we all, big, small or microscopic, have to contend with?"

"Gravity."

"Exactly. You learn fast, Carter. Gravity has an affect on

every living thing on this planet. And opposition to gravity is the common denominator of all exercises."

"Hold it. Are you saying that opposition to gravity is the very essence of exercise?"

"Certainly. There has to be an opposing force to work against in order to develop strength. Gravity is a universal physical constant, the downward pull which all living things must contend with. Check it out, Carter. When you do pushups, what are you pushing away from?"

"Gravity."

"Right. In the activities classified as aerobic exercise, such as walking, jogging, and running, you humans lean forward slightly in response to gravity's pull, then oppose gravity by taking a step."

"You're right, Larry. Walking, jogging, and running have all been defined as a state of continuous falling, almost falling over, but not quite. But what about swimming? I float. That sort of cancels out gravity, doesn't it?"

"You're not exercising when you're floating, Carter, only when you're actually swimming. It's atmospheric pressure which holds water in place and compresses it sufficiently to make it dense enough so that you have a force to oppose when you swim. The earth's atmosphere is held in place by gravity as well," he explained patiently.

"Of course," I agreed. "And it's easy to see that weight-lifting works against gravity. The effectiveness of weight-lifting equates to mass-times-gravity. You lift a mass away from the pull of gravity in order to exercise certain muscles."

"Humans do, Carter. Cells don't."

"Sorry. I just got carried away with the logic behind this conversation."

"Cells are carried away. You, Carter, are held in your chair in front of your word processor by gravity. What do you suppose would happen to you if you were subjected to a 2-G force, that's twice the force of normal earth gravity, for an extended period of time?"

"Theoretically, I guess I would become twice as strong. All living organisms have the ability to react to changes in their environment."

"What would happen to all of the 75 trillion cells that make up your body?"

"You guys would become stronger, too."

"There you have it."

"Oh, sure, Larry," I mocked. "All we have to do is manage somehow to beef up the pull of gravity to 2-Gs."

"Or fool your cells into believing that you have that power," he shot back.

"This is beginning to sound like science-fiction, Larry."

"More like science-*fact*, Carter. As early as 1911, Albert Einstein presented a new fact about gravity. Einstein said that the forces of acceleration and deceleration have the same effects on the human body as gravity does. This information became very important as time went on because NASA scientists had to know in advance exactly how much G-force the astronauts could withstand in space flight before they started falling apart from the strain."

"Then our scientists know all about the effects of acceleration and deceleration on the human body, right?"

"Not exactly. You see, NASA was only interested in determining what acceleration during liftoff would do to the human body, and what amount of stress deceleration would cause to the body during reentry into the earth's atmosphere. They never considered the peripheral health benefits that small controlled spurts of acceleration and deceleration could offer to the human organism."

"What's the best way to apply these two forces?"

"Vertically. Line them up with gravity."

"That would mean jumping up and down," I answered.

"Not good enough, Carter. You'd come to a deadstop on landing. Rebounding on your rebound exercise thing is the

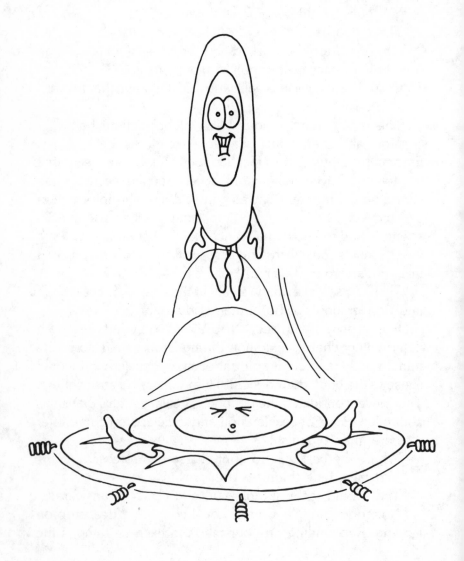

answer."

"Oh, that. You mean The Dyna-Bound. I've been using it to run-in-place indoors. I never thought of just jumping up and down on it."

"It's very good for running or jogging, Carter. I approve. Rebounding on that springy, resilient pad eliminates as much as seven-eighths of the shock-trauma to the joints of your feet and ankles that occurs when you perform the same movements outdoors. Incidentally, I like this trampoline much better than the one you had before."

"I do, too, Larry. But what difference does it make to you?" I asked, curious to see what he would say.

"The other one didn't have much spring to it, Carter. Besides, you gave all of us an awful jolt the day one of those spindly legs collapsed and dumped you on the floor. This one gives us all a really good workout. It must be better. What's the difference between the two anyway?"

"The Dyna-Bound is very well made, Larry." I answered, glad to find myself in a position where I knew more than he did for once. "The pad is genuine Permatron, which insures more bounce to the ounce. The Dyna-Bound's triangulated springs are made of #80 carbon steel wire to reduce breakage. Health Energy Products, the manufacturer, says I can expect almost lifetime service from this one. Another thing I really like is that when NASA tested rebounding, they selected The Dyna-Bound as the best rebound exerciser on the market. NASA says, when you use quality equipment, rebounding is 68 percent more efficient than jogging. The Dyna-Bound folds in the middle, and its legs fold down, too. It fits in its own carrying case, so I can easily take it with me when I travel. Or I can fold it up and pop it in its case for dust-free storage."

"Oh, no! Don't store it away, Carter."

"Why not?"

"As I told you before, rebounding is the only kind of exercise that we cells can really appreciate. Remember a few minutes ago when we were talking about the force of gravity? When you rebound every day, every cell in your body gets stronger, and so do you. In order for the cells of your lymphatic system to receive the full benefit of exercise, it's necessary for you to alter our environment by increasing the G-force."

"And rebounding does that?"

"You bet it does. When you're standing still, every cell in your body is subjected to one G-force. But when you jump up and down vertically on The Dyna-Bound, you are adding two other forces. . ."

"Acceleration and deceleration." I finished the sentence for him.

"Exactly. The combination of all three forces - gravity, acceleration and deceleration - subjects all the cells in your body to increased G-force. We cells don't know that you're increasing the G-force by rebounding. We can't tell the difference, you see. But we adjust quickly to the increased G-force in our environment, which you create when you rebound. We become stronger and stronger."

"Come on, Larry. Everybody knows that exercise strengthens muscles. But are you really saying that rebounding is a *cellular* exercise?" I questioned. "It's hard to believe that something so simple - and so much fun - can work so well."

"Rebounding works spectacularly, Carter. You have a copy of *The Miracles of Rebound Exercise*, don't you?"

"Sure. But that's an old book. It was published back in the late 1970's, I believe."

"That's true. But what I wanted to point out is that '*Miracles*' is full of stories of real people who say that rebounding regularly has improved their health immeasurably and changed their lives for the better. Don't you remember reading about them?"

"I guess I do remember, now that you mention it. Some of those people were really sick before they started rebounding. Even so, that book can't be very up-to-date. After 10 years, there must be a lot more current information on rebounding by now."

"Oh, there is. That's why the world's foremost authority on rebounding is putting out a second edition. *The New Miracles of Rebound Exercise* contains all the information that was in the first one, plus a whole lot more."

"Like what, Larry?"

"Well, Carter," he sounded very pleased, "I'm glad to say that your scientists are finally coming around to my way of thinking. Finnish researchers compared fifty runners and cross-country skiers who each jogged about 30 miles per week to fifty healthy men who didn't exercise. They found that those who trained consistently had thicker, more flexible skin tissue."

"So? Any program of regular exercise can accomplish that."

"Right. But remember, please, that the common denominator of all forms of exercise is opposition to gravity. We cells begin responding immediately to a change in gravity. In just fourteen days of spaceflight at zero gravity, your astronauts lost 15 percent of their bone and muscle mass, Carter." He hammered home his point. "Rats lost 40 percent in only seven days."

"That's bone and muscle mass, Larry. I don't believe our medical scientists had anything to say about space-hopping lymphocytes."

"No, not your U.S. scientists. But human astronauts aren't the only space travelers that researchers abroad are interested in. A scientific study by seven scientists representing four different laboratories in Switzerland has revealed that lymphocytes extracted from U.S. astronauts and Russian cosmonauts were as much as 15 percent less active after spaceflight, all because they had adjusted to a zero gravity environmemt."

"So, logically speaking, all live cells in a zero gravity situation adjust by becoming weaker."

"Of course we do. And, if you still doubt that every living organism adjusts to environmental changes, here's the clincher.

The Swiss scientists subjected those same white blood cells to an increase of 4-G's. After only three days, they found that the cells had plumped up and exhibited richer vacuols, an unusually high quantity of mitochondria, and were as much as five times more active."

"Meaning that the cells were bioelectrically more potent than normal cells at 1-G. That is impressive." I was getting really interested in the concept of cellular exercise. "So, Larry, if I subject my two-pound army of lymphocytes to an increased G-force environment 100 times per minute, all you guys will become individually stronger and more potent. Collectively, my immune defense forces can become invincible!"

"That's what you want, isn't it?"

"Of course! Everyone should be rebounding!"

"That's one of the reasons why we're writing this book, Carter. But there's still more for you to learn."

"How can there be?"

"You humans need to know that rebounding is the most efficient way of activating the first-line defenders of your body, the entire lymphatic system."

"Why is that?" I asked, genuinely interested.

"Because, just like the veins of your cardiovascular system, the veins and passageways of the lymphatic system are filled with millions of one-way valves to insure that the lymph flows upward toward the heart."

"Why is that so important?"

"That's our main way of traveling. Have you forgotten the tour I took you on so soon? After we leave the bloodstream through the pores in the capillaries, we move through the tissues and finally find our way to a lymphatic terminal, where we are sucked into the lymph veins along with metabolic trash and toxins. Your lymphatic system is not directly connected to the heart, Carter, so we don't have a beating muscle to push us along. The only way we can circulate is through the one-way valves that bar the way. When we reach a valve, it must be activated for us to continue making rounds. Vigorous rebounding can increase your lymph flow from 15 to 30-fold, making our job of cleaning up your body many times more efficient."

"Wow! If rebounding provides me with a stronger army that can patrol much faster, I can see how rebounding might be classified as an incredible cancer-deterrent."

"Wait! There's still more."

"Now you're beginning to sound like a television commercial, Larry."

"Don't digress, Carter. Pay attention here," he said sternly. "You have a standing army of 5,000 neutrophils for every cubic millimeter of blood in your body when you're healthy. That army increases to as many as 25,000 within just a few hours of any sign of inflammation or a foreign invader."

"That's very comforting to know," I acknowledged.

"If we immune system cells identify cancer, the number of neutrophils ready to protect you will increase to as many as three-times the normal number."

"Nothing takes the place of good security," I remarked.

"But you don't have to wait for an attack from a foreign invader or cancer to appear on the scene, Carter. You can call out the troops at a moment's notice any time of the day or night."

"How do I do that?"

"You seem to put a lot of stock in your medical authorities, Carter. Do you have a copy of *Medical Physiology* handy?"

"Sure do. Right here on my desk," I answered.

"Good. Open it up to page 57 and read halfway down the right-hand column."

"Do you have this book memorized, Larry?"

"Only as much as you do," he answered. "Read!"

"I'm reading! I'm reading:

'The number of neutrophils in the circulatory system can increase to as much as two to three times normal after a single minute of extremely hard exercise.'

"So, if I get on The Dyna-Bound and run-in-place just as fast as I can for just one minute, three-times as many white blood cells will be called out to look for foreign invaders and mutant cells. Is that right, Larry?"

"Either that, or your book is incorrect."

"Wow! How long will these extra soldiers remain on patrol?"

"Read the last paragraph of that same section."

"Okay:

'Approximately one hour after physiological neutrophilia has resulted from exercise, the number of neutrophils in the blood is usually back to normal.' "

"By now, Carter, I'm sure you're beginning to see why scientists at Harvard University found that less active women had a two and one-half times greater risk of developing cancer than did the former athletes among them. These preventable types of cancer account for more than 40 percent of all cancers in women. These results grew out of a study of over 5,000 female students who graduated from ten U.S. colleges between 1925 and 1981."

"So the bottom line is that by a combination of cell-food and cell-exercise, we humans can help you soldiers of our immune defense forces to become considerably more proficient in your work."

"Very definitely, Carter. But, wait! There's still more."

"You've been watching too many television commercials, Larry," I said with a smile.

He ignored my quip. "Plus the combination of cell-food and cell-exercise, add in cell-environment, Carter."

"That sounds like a good idea, little buddy. I'm thirsty. Here's a cup of cell-environment coming up."

"You mean 'coming down,' Carter."

I smiled to myself at his quick correction. He was beginning to remind me more and more of another fan of logic and precisely accurate speech, Mr. Spock, the imaginary Vulcan of *Star Trek* fame.

"I'm going to take a swim now, Larry. I need to cool off. Don't you have something important to do?"

"Unlike you humans, I always have something *important* to do, Carter," he said tartly. "I guess humans can't be expected to be on duty 24 hours a day, as we are. I know you find a dip in the pool refreshing, but we cells like it better when you rebound. By the way Carter, why don't you tell the reader where he might find the Dyna-Bound and *The New Miracles* book."

I didn't bother answering this time. I knew he was determined to have the last word, so I just started typing.

The Dyna-Bound and *The New Miracles* can usually be found in local health food stores, but if unavailable there, you can contact the company directly as follows:

New Dimensions Distributors, Inc.
16548 E. Laser Drive, Suite A-7
Fountain Hills, AZ 85268
1-800-624-7114   Toll-Free Nationwide
1-602-837-8322   In Arizona

Bibliography

Carter, AE: The Miracles of Rebound Exercise. Edmonds, WA: The National Institute of Reboundology and Health, 1979.

Guyton, AC: Text Book of Medical Physiology. Philadelphia: WB Saunders Co, 1986.

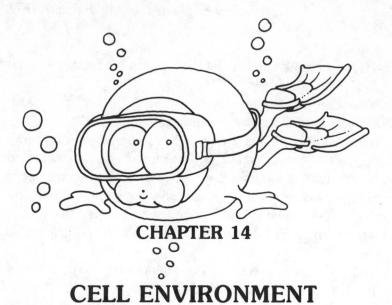

CHAPTER 14

CELL ENVIRONMENT

"Come on, kids. Out of the pool," my wife Bonnie called, letting us know dinner was ready. I love it when she includes me in the term 'kids.' Just to make sure I wouldn't lose my status, I splashed my daughter Melynda a few more times before I backstroked into the shallow end and climbed out.

"Oh, my!" Bonnie exclaimed. "Go look in the mirror. Your eyes are all red."

"I can imagine," I agreed. "It's the chlorine in the pool. It always makes my eyes bloodshot. I'm glad I don't have to live in there. I can only stand so much of it before my eyes really begin to sting."

I inhaled deeply. It was much easier to breathe without pool water being splashed in my face. 'Life is good,' I thought as I grabbed a fluffy oversized towel and began to wipe the water off my face. I walked over to the inviting buffet that Bonnie had prepared.

Since my shopping expedition with Larry, we had discovered that there is a real difference between 'people food' and cell-food.' We had found with pleasure that the best-tasting foods were those which also qualified as cell-food. The salad bar

Bonnie had laid out was rich with foods capable of tantalizing the taste buds with their own special signatures of chemical differences. The salt and white sugar which had masked the natural flavors of foods were no longer part of our diet. We seemed to have a lot more energy, fewer headaches, and no more sniffles. 'Thank you, Larry,' I thought to myself.

"You're welcome, Carter," I heard in answer. "Now, do yourself a favor."

"What's that?" I asked aloud.

"That's potato and spinach salad, dear, topped with a sprinkle of bee pollen granules," Bonnie answered.

"I'm sorry, Bonnie. I was talking to Larry."

"Oh, how sweet!" she exclaimed. "What's he telling you this time?"

"I don't know - yet."

"Well, you just go ahead and talk to him if you want to. We'll understand." She turned away and said, "Children, don't bother Daddy. He's talking to Larry again."

"This is embarrassing," I muttered under my breath.

"Don't blame me, Carter," Larry said promptly. "I didn't tell you to tell them about me."

"I had to, Larry. They couldn't figure out where I was getting all my information."

"Don't they believe in inspiration?"

"Not this kind. Not for a whole book."

"Carter, why don't you excuse yourself and go to your word processor?"

"I haven't eaten yet," I protested. "And it's all good cell food..."

"You can last forty days without eating. You won't starve."

"It might come as a surprise to you, little buddy, but I *like* to eat."

"No surprise, Carter. In fact, I've been meaning to talk to you about that."

"About what?"

"Your excess food intake."

"I've been eating good food."

"I know. Good food, but too much and too often. You can get fat even on good food ."

"Look, Larry, I don't tell you what to eat, or how much."

"Until very recently, Carter, you didn't give me much of a choice. I had to figure out how to get rid of all the garbage you were dishing in."

"That's not happening now, Larry," I said earnestly. "I don't eat what you call 'garbage' any longer. I shop for cell-food. I've even taught my family how to identify cell-food, and they love it, too. You'll have to admit that we have eliminated all the bad chemicals from our diet."

"I wish I could, Carter, because we'd both be much healthier if you had."

"Okay, Larry. I'll go to my word processor. But, I'm warning you, this had better be good. I hope you realize that I'm depriving the cells of my taste buds the privilege of the neural excitation they get when sorting out and distinguishing the various flavors of the fruits and vegetables awaiting my palate."

"You almost make me wish I was a human, Carter. But, believe me, we are doing this book for our own good."

I was still hungry. "Okay, Larry, if you're determined to save the world... "

"Just *my* world," he interrupted. "You are my whole world."

"Point well taken. I just get a little on edge when I'm hungry."

"I don't fault you for that, Carter. Hunger is a mechanism designed to keep us healthy."

I gave up. "Okay, oh mighty cytotoxic T cell. Here I am at the word processor, as you ordered. Speak!"

"Before we begin, go look at yourself in the mirror," he instructed.

"I know. My eyes are all bloodshot and they look terrible. That happens whenever I swim in the pool."

"Why do you suppose that happens, Carter?"

"Too much chlorine, I guess. No biggie. It goes away eventually."

He refused to be sidetracked. "How much chlorine is too much?"

"Enough to make my eyes bloodshot." I was getting irritated. "What is this? Twenty questions?"

"Why do you put chlorine in your swimming pool?"

I sighed. "To kill germs and bacteria, of course."

"Does it work?"

"Of course it works. Chlorine is a well-known germicide. We even used chlorine gas in the first World War to kill our enemies."

"Do you know how chlorine works as a germ killer?"

"I never really gave it much thought."

"Chlorine upsets the electrical potential of the cell membrane. The chloride ion is highly soluble in water and diffuses rapidly through cell membranes," he explained. "Because it's so potent, we cells use it inside the body in assisting in the maintenance of the normal electrolyte balance in all your tissues. We also use it to produce hydrochloric acid in your stomach for digestive purposes."

"I think what you're saying in your precise way is that adding chlorine to swimming pool water produces so many positive ions that bacteria can't live in that environment."

"Right. Let's find out how well your memory is functioning, Carter. What are bacteria and germs?"

"They are 'bad cells,' foreign invaders."

"Does chlorine kill them?"

"Yes."

"Then chlorine is a known cell-killer?"

"You bet. One of the best."

Can you figure out why your eyes are so bloodshot?"

I was beginning to put it together. "Because I have just killed millions of cells of my eyes."

"What about the cells of the rest of your body?"

"I guess it will kill many of them also," I answered slowly.

"Very good, Carter," he approved sarcastically. "Do you suppose that's why many swimmers develop skin rashes?"

"I guess so," I answered reluctantly.

"If you want to put chlorine in your human pool, I guess that's up to you. We cells will still try to keep you healthy. But, Carter, is it absolutely necessary to put that known cell-killer in *my* pool?"

He had me mystified now. "I don't put chlorine in your pool, Larry."

"Where do you get the water you drink?"

"From the tap, of course," I answered promptly.

"How does your municipal water supplier keep the bacterial population of the water under control?"

"They add chlorine to the water and it kills the bad cells."

"Not only the *bad* cells, Carter. Do you suppose the killing stops at your lips?"

"No, Larry. . ." I was suddenly shocked. "I'm sorry. I never thought much about it."

"You're not the only one, Carter. Most humans don't think about the problems their water can cause. Every time a cell dies, it becomes the responsibility of the immune system defense forces to clean up the mess. That type of *unnecessary* activity reduces the efficiency of our main *fighting* abilities."

"You're telling me that you can't do two things at once, right?"

"Or be in two places at once."

"That makes two things that humans and cells have in common."

"We have more in common than that, Carter. On average, you consume 2,300 milliliters of water per day, and get rid of the same amount."

"Impossible! That equals nine cups! I don't drink nine cups of water any day - even when I swim"

"True, you don't *drink* that much water, Carter. Only

two-thirds of your intake is in the form of water, or some other beverage. The remainder is in the food you eat, with the exception of about one cup, or 250 milliliters. We distill that much water inside your body by oxidizing the hydrogen out of some of the foods you eat."

"Clever."

"Yes, I think so. It would be nice, Carter, if we could get *all* our water that way. Then we wouldn't have to defend against all the pollutants in the water you drink," he said forcefully.

I filed that information away for discussion later. I was still wondering what happened to the nine cups of water Larry assured me I took in every day. "I suppose you can tell me how I get rid of 2,300 milliliters of water every day?"

"Simple, Carter. You breathe out approximately 350 milliliters, and another 350 milliliters disappears through your skin."

"As sweat?"

"No. This is moisture lost by diffusion right through your skin cells. We don't need the sweat glands to process that much. At normal body temperature, you may lose around 100 milliliters by sweating. In hot weather, you could lose up to 1,400 milliliters through your sweat glands."

"How much could I lose if I exercised for a long period of time in hot weather?"

"You could lose up to 6,600 milliliters of water, with 5,000 of the total amount as sweat," he answered quickly.

I did a quick calculation. "Wow! That's over 26 cups of water in one day! Larry, that adds up to almost seven quarts of water lost!"

"I didn't say it was *healthy*, Carter. I said you'd lose that much during prolonged heavy exercise in hot weather. But that would seriously upset homeostasis in here. If you were competing in an endurance athletic event under hot and humid conditions, you could lose up to ten pounds of weight in one hour. Almost all that weight loss could be attributed to sweating, because of the excessive buildup of body heat."

"Body heat? Where would all that heat come from?" I asked curiously.

"On our very best days, we can only convert 20 to 25 percent of your nutrient energy stores into muscle energy. The rest is converted into heat," he explained patiently. "If you were to exercise as hard as you can, you could possibly increase your oxygen consumption by twenty times. The body heat liberated in exercise is directly proportional to the amount of oxygen you use. Your body heat would increase from a comfortable 98.6 degrees F. to as high as a deadly 108 degrees. The combination of extreme body heat and loss of body water can be devastating to all the cells of your body."

"Are you talking about a heat stroke, Larry?"

"I'm talking about a major emergency, you dunderhead!" he said witheringly. "Major groups of cells would stop functioning. The control mechanisms would send out the wrong signals. Cells would be dying."

"I know the symptoms, Larry. Weakness, exhaustion, headache, dizziness, nausea, profuse sweating, staggering, collapse, unconsciousness, and even death. But neither one of us has to worry about that. I'm not going to go out and run a marathon, I assure you."

He calmed down a little. "Carter, I wonder if you know just how much effort your cells expend in order to control the internal environment of your body."

"What do you mean?"

"Well, do you heat your human pool?"

"No."

"We do. Do you measure the level of ions in the air you breathe?"

"Of course not."

"We do. And how about the quantity and quality of the food you eat? Do you monitor that?"

"I've never found it necessary, Larry."

"That's right. You didn't find any of those things necessary because we've been doing them for you. You see, Professor, the internal environment of your body can't be taken lightly. It's the home of your more than 75 trillion cells. By weight, 57 percent of your body is water. When you were a baby, your water-weight tallied as high as 75 percent. Just before you die, the water content of your body can be as low as 45 percent. Remember, Carter, about 25 percent of your 40 liters of water is inside your 75 trillion cells."

"Scientifically known as intracellular fluid, protoplasm or cytoplasm," I contributed.

"We live in the other 15 liters."

"And that's known in scientific terminology as extracellular fluid, interstitial fluid, or the internal environment," I interjected.

"We cells depend on the constant mix of your body fluids to supply us with the water, oxygen, hormones, and nutrients we need to function. There's three times as much extracellular fluid in your body as there is blood. Carter, water is more important to life than all nutrients combined."

"Now wait a minute, Larry. That's hard to believe. You cells need good food just as much as I do. Water can't be more important."

"On the contrary, Carter. You think of water as something to quench your thirst. But we cells need water for every cellular activity we perform. Water is critical to efficient kidney function and waste removal. Water is required to control your body temperature. It is also an absolutely essential solvent and the transport system for many nutrients, including some important vitamins you can't live without. Water lubricates your digestive tract, and cushions your joints. It is an essential part of the protective systems of your eyes, both inside and out. You probably know that blood is almost all water, but did you know that your bones are more than 20 percent water?"

He had me. "Frankly, no," I admitted. "All I remember being taught is that my water intake should be replenished in accordance with the demands I make on my body. In a stressed situation, such as a demanding 10K run or a hike across the desert, I know that my body will use up water much faster than normal. In order to guard against potentially dangerous dehydration, it's vitally important that water intake be adjusted to the level of activity."

"So far, so good, Carter. And keep in mind that water is the universal solvent. It can get through all of your cell membranes in order to take nutrients in, or waste material and hormones out."

"Okay, you've made your point," I conceded. "The cells of my body need water. But is it possible to get too much of a good thing? Can I take in too much water?"

"Definitely. In a normal individual, the intake and output of water are in a state of equilibrium, and the individual is technically termed in a state of 'water-balance.' But taking in water in excess of the ability of the body to eliminate water may produce a state of 'water intoxication.' "

"I have plenty of beer-drinking friends who would laugh at that statement, Larry," I said with a smile.

He ignored my observation. "But not drinking enough fluids can also be devastating, Carter. Dehydration, a water loss exceeding your water intake by just 10 percent, can result in illness. Losing 20 percent can result in death."

I got serious again. "Okay, let me get this straight, Larry. If I drink too *much* water, or don't drink *enough* water, I'm in trouble either way. I have to drink just enough to be A-OK. Right?"

"Carter, for both our sakes, I wish that was so. Unfortunately, drinking the water that comes into your home and flows out of your tap may be the greatest source of all the cancer-inducing agents to which you and your family are exposed."

I smiled tolerantly. "I know, Larry. That's why chlorine is added to our water supply."

"Chlorine's adding to the problem, Carter. Go eat your

cell-food now. When you're finished stuffing your face, take a trip to the library and find out all you can about chlorine."

"Okay," I answered agreeably. "I'll go tonight right after dinner."

"And, while you're at it, Carter, see what you can find about fluoride, too."

"You mean that stuff they put in toothpaste to prevent cavities?"

"And in your water supply for the same purpose, Carter."

It took me two days of intensive digging into published scientific research reports on water and what ends up in it before I was satisfied. Unfortunately, I found I was even more confused than I was before Larry got on his soapbox.

"Larry."

"Yes, Carter?"

"This is all very confusing."

"Actually, since you did all that extensive reading at the library over the past two days, it has become much clearer to me."

"Thank heavens! If it's clearer to you, I wish you'd share your insights with me."

"Simple. We cells follow the strict rules of the body, or we face elimination. These rules were established thousands of years ago and are based on true principles. But many times, humans - and your greatest scientists are human - follow a group of rules dictated by 'politics.' Too often, these rules have absolutely no regard for truth."

I winced. "Larry, that statement is so harsh that I don't think we should include it in this book at all."

"I'm just getting started, Carter. Don't hold me back! Do you remember everything you've read during the past two days?"

"Most of it, I think. For example, most community water systems supply heavily chlorinated water which they say is purified and which is considered to be of acceptable potable, or drinking quality. And a great many community water systems also routinely add fluoride as a decay preventive to the drinking water they deliver to local homes."

"Okay, Carter. Let's take them one at a time. Start with chlorine. Did you find out what it is"

"I think so. Chlorine is a nonmetallic element, a diatomic gas that is heavy, noncombustible, and greenish-yellow. It has a pungent irritating odor. In liquid form, it is a clear amber color, also with an irritating odor. It is toxic and irritating to skin and lungs."

"Where is it found?"

"It doesn't occur in a free state, but is a component of the mineral halite, better known as rock salt."

"What are some of its uses?"

"Chlorine is used in the manufacture of carbon tetrachloride and trichlorethylene, for water purification, and in shrink-proofing wool. It's put in flame retardant compounds, and used in processing fish, vegetables, and fruit."

"Okay, Carter. Why do you suppose chlorine is used to process fish, vegetables, and fruit."

"Probably because it does a good job of killing bacteria and other things that would cause fresh foods to rot."

"We have already established the fact that chlorine is an effective cell poison, but there's something overlooked by your human water purification experts."

"What's that?"

"The chlorine used to kill bacteria in water often contains carbon tetrachloride, a contaminant formed during the production process."

"Yes, I caught that, too. The Environmental Protection Agency points out that carbon tetrachloride has been inadvertently added to drinking water in Philadelphia and many other cities. Pretty scary."

"What's the Environmental Protection Agency, Carter?"

"It's a political organization developed for the purpose of improving our environment. They're charged with the responsibility of looking after the interests of the consumer."

"Oh, sure," he said with a trace of sarcasm. "And what did you find out about carbon tetrachloride?"

"Carbon tet is a colorless, clear, nonflammable, heavy liquid obtained from carbon disulfide and chlorine. It's used in fire extinguishers, for dry-cleaning clothes, for rendering benzene nonflammable, as a drying agent for wet spark plugs in automobiles, as a solvent for oils, fats, lacquers, varnishes, rubber, waxes, resins, and for exterminating insects, including hookworms and tape worms," I answered.

"Gross and disgusting! And this stuff is in your *drinking* water?"

"Only *inadvertently,* Larry." I emphasized that point. "It's poisonous by inhalation, ingestion, or skin absorption. They certainly don't put it in on purpose, you know."

"You're talking sudden destruction, Carter. Acute carbon tetrachloride poisoning causes nausea, diarrhea, headaches, stupor, kidney damage, and death."

He had my full attention. "This is serious."

"It certainly is 'serious.' Carbon tetrachloride has caused cancer in rats, mice, and hamsters when given orally, subcutaneously, and rectally."

"That sounds bad," I acknowledged.

"Maybe your EPA can do something about the fact that chlorinating water has also been known to cause the formation of other undesirable chemical compounds in water, such as toluene, xylene, and styrene."

"Are these compounds harmful, Larry?"

"To the cells of your body, they're deadly. They kill off red and white blood cells, destroy skin cells, and produce serious heart problems."

"I guess that makes it easier to understand those research reports I read which show there's a 44 percent higher incidence of gastro-intestinal and urinary tract cancers in populations drinking chlorinated water than in matching control groups drinking non-chlorinated water." I sighed. "The saddest thing of all, Larry, is that most public water supply systems use chlorine to disinfect water, and these chemicals are present in virtually every water supply tested by the EPA."

"Does all this tell you anything, Carter?"

"Yes. I shouldn't be drinking water from the tap."

"We're not finished yet. Have you heard of chloroform?"

"Of course."

"Chloroform has caused cancer in test animals. Can you tell me why it would produce the same effect in humans?"

I had learned my lesson well. "Because it reduces the effectiveness of the immune system by poisoning you lymphocytes, and by killing other cells, thereby overburdening my immune defense forces."

"Why?"

"Because you lymphocytes also are assigned the job of ingesting all those dead cells. You and your cousins would be seriously overworked and wouldn't have time to clean up the mutant cells that turn into cancer."

"Congratulations, Carter. You are beginning to understand. So, is chlorine a safe bactericide?"

"No."

"True, chlorine does destroy the waterborne bacteria which causes typhoid fever, cholera, and dysentery. But chlorine injures red blood cells and damages their ability to carry life-giving oxygen where it's needed."

"Here's something you'll be interested in, Larry. Over 10 years ago, U.S.S.R. scientists discovered that people drinking water containing 1.4 milligrams ppm (parts per million) of chlorine had higher blood pressure readings on average than those drinking water with only .3 to .4 milligrams ppm of chlorine."

"That spells arterial cellular destruction, Carter. That means the immune system defense forces are required to repair the damage by scabbing, which, in turn, causes arterial chloresterol buildup, resulting in an obstruction. That makes it harder for the heart to pump blood, accounting for the increase in blood pressure."

"That sounds like a reasonable explanation," I acknowledged.

"Factual," he answered tersely.

"Here's another bit of news, Larry. As long ago as 1973, patients undergoing kidney dialysis at two artificial kidney centers in the U.S. uniformly developed severe anemia. Laboratory studies ferreted out the cause. Chlorinated water was being used in the dialysis machines. When the chlorine damaged red blood cells, those unfortunate patients developed serious anemia."

"I'm not surprised, Carter. That adds up to still more evidence that chlorine is a proven cell poison."

"Well, Larry, if I *have* to drink chlorinated water, the good news is that science has discovered an inexpensive way to neutralize the chlorine. A tiny pinch of ascorbic acid powder, vitamin C, in a glass of water will neutralize the chlorine and protect my red blood cells from injury. The vitamin C will erase the taste and eliminate the characteristic odor as well. My water will taste better, too."

"Always thinking of yourself, aren't you, Carter? The bad news is that merely neutralizing the chlorine is not enough to guarantee the water you drink is safe for me. There are a lot more pollutants in your water than the obvious ones that chlorine kills," he said vehemently.

"What do you mean, Larry?"

"The drinking water that comes into your home is probably the source of the greatest number of cancer-inducing agents that you put into your body. There are literally thousands of organic chemicals potentially present in the water supplies of your nation due to industrial discharges and spills, the use of agricultural chemicals, and the runoff of dirty and contaminated rainwater from cities. Where do most humans get their drinking water, Carter?"

"Let's see." I consulted my notes. "It says here that most municipal water supplies come from groundwater."

"What's groundwater?"

"That's subsurface water which supplies springs, lakes, and rivers. Groundwater supplies 20 percent of the fresh water used in the United States. It constitutes the entire water supply of more than 95 percent of the rural population, and 20 percent of the one hundred largest cities in the country. The semi-arid Southwest is almost completely dependent on groundwater.

"Groundwater can be polluted by dirty surface water sinking down and mingling with it, deep well disposal systems, seepage from mines, landfills, septic tanks, feed lots, and agricultural chemicals and pesticides. It is estimated that 10 million barrels of brine are injected into underground reservoirs by the gas and oil industries every year."

"Carter, we're in big trouble. I can't control what you drink. I just have to wait until it enters your body before I can try to deal with it."

"I think you might be right, Larry," I replied. "Our human scientists admit they know relatively little about the chemicals that pollute our water supplies. But they know that many of these chemicals do create an internal environment favorable to cancer in test animals."

For the first time, he sounded discouraged. "Isn't there any hope of help?"

"The wheels grind slowly in the real world, Larry. The Safe Drinking Water Act enacted in 1974 required that the administrator of the EPA work with the National Academy of Sciences in mounting a study to determine the safety of our drinking water. The academy's 1975 study revealed thousands of organic chemicals in the drinking water of 80 cities. The committee determined that volatile organic compounds make up 10 percent by weight of the total organic matter in water.

"They examined 74 nonpesticides from among the more than 300 volatile organic compounds identified. They also examined 55 pesticides, some of which were not detected in water at that time, but which they surmised would be expected to show up because of their widespread use. They judged 22 of these compounds to be either known carcinogens, or suspected carcinogens, for both humans and animals. The NAS committee noted that chlorination, the primary control of waterborne infections, may result in the formation of suspected carcinogens for humans, and proposed substitute disinfectants for our water supplies."

"Carter, there are a discouraging number of chemicals today which you are introducing into my home, your internal environment, that we must defend against, and which we have never before experienced."

"I know, Larry," I said sympathetically. "The widespread contamination of our environment by synthetic chemicals is a relatively recent development in the scheme of things. The lifetime exposure of the human population to these chemicals poses a serious threat to public heath, including an increased risk of cancer."

"You got that right, Carter." He pulled himself together. I pictured him squaring his nonexistent shoulders before he continued. "Now tell me about fluorine."

I corrected him. "You mean *fluoride,* Larry. That's the stuff that goes in water and toothpaste to prevent cavities."

"I wish you humans would make up your mind. In Europe, they call it 'fluor.' But in the English speaking countries, you can't seem to decide whether it should be called fluorine or fluoride."

"My toothpaste says FLUORIDE in big red letters," I explained helpfully.

"Chemically speaking, Carter, it should be called fluorine because it's one of the halogen group of chemicals. The other three are chlorine, bromine, and iodine."

"That makes sense. The true chemists probably do call it fluorine."

"Using the 'n' would clarify just what we're discussing. For example, if a human were to ingest 1 milligram of sodium fluoride, approximately 45 percent of it would be fluorine, and the rest would be sodium. However, I notice that even your medical experts are extremely vague on which term to use."

"Who cares? What difference does it make anyway?"

"Carter, if we are talking about a possibly lethal dose of poison, wouldn't you want to know if it was twice as deadly, or only half a death-dealing dose?"

"If we were talking about a *poison*, Larry, of course. But this stuff is put into our water supply to keep us from having cavities. It's not poison."

"And you tell me humans are supposed to possess superior intelligence, Carter," he said witheringly.

"Look, Larry, you don't have teeth. You don't know what it's like to suffer a toothache because of a cavity, or to make repeated trips to a dentist to get your cavities filled. Our scientists have found an economical way to fight cavities for the entire population of the United States, and many other countries have followed suit as well."

"Okay, my good man." I could tell by his voice that he had adopted the role of 'teacher' again. "I'm doing this for the health of both of us. Tell me all you know about fluoride."

"Fluoride is an acid salt they put in toothpaste and our water supplies to prevent tooth decay," I answered promptly.

"That's it? Nothing else?"

"What else do I need to know?"

"Carter, the plain truth is that fluorine is an insidious poison. It's toxic, very harmful, and cumulative in effect. Even when ingested in minimal amounts, fluorine remains in the tissues and builds up over time. No matter how many sources call it 'safe,' the fact remains that fluorine is one of the poisons we have to try to defend you against."

"There you go again, Larry," I scolded. "You're making claims you can't back up. The American Dental Association supports fluoridation. So does the American Medical Association, the Food & Drug Administration, and the World Health Organization, plus about every other health organization you can name."

"Yup. And because these humans endorse it, that means it's OK. Right?"

"They're the experts, Larry."

"Humans have a saying that fits, Carter. 'The blind leading the blind.' "

"You don't have eyes, Larry. You're really blind."

"Nonetheless, Carter, I can see what fluorine is doing to some of my fellow cells. They just happen to be part of the same body I inhabit, and that body just happens to be yours."

"Okay, Larry. Riddle me this: If fluoride is so bad for us, why do our health experts endorse fluoridation of our drinking water?"

"That's what *I'm* asking *you*, Carter. But I think I have the answer. It's because of ignorance, pride, greed, and politics. All of which are human frailties."

"You don't like politics, do you, Larry?"

"Carter, politics are an imprecise method of establishing rules and regulations for organisms capable of ruling themselves. As I said before, sometimes these regulations are not based on truth."

"Is that so bad, Larry? Humans need rules and regulations. As long as everyone lives by the same rules, what harm can come from it?"

"If decisions are based on politics instead of truth, it will be devastating to the humans who are depending on their experts when the truth is finally revealed, Carter," he said patiently. "For example, ever since your politicans and scientists endorsed fluoridation, they have been forced to defend it in the face of increasing worldwide opposition from many responsible scientists. As a result, the reputation of your dental organizations and other health organizations have become irrevocably bound to the fate of fluoridation. You humans have now reached the stage where rejecting water fluoridation and the direct treating of teeth with fluoride will irreparably discredit the American Dental Association and the related research published by the U.S. Public Health Service."

"Do you really think the fluoridation program has something to do with politics, Larry?"

"You tell me. Where did you humans get the idea that fluoride prevents cavities?"

"Back in the 1930s, H. Trendley Dean of the U.S. Public Health Service was engaged in investigating the effects of naturally-occurring fluoride. He noted a connection between mottled teeth and an absence of dental caries, or cavities. Dean is now popularly known as the 'Father of Fluoridation.' "

"What do you mean by mottled teeth, Carter?"

"The term 'mottled enamel' to describe discolored teeth appears to have made its first appearance in medical literature in 1915. But dark spots on teeth were written about as early as 1771. In 1878 one medical writer said, '. . . White, yellow, or brown spots of various sizes and irregular shapes may exist on outer surfaces of the teeth. . . Sometimes, several of the teeth in one or both jaws may be so severely affected as to scarcely look like teeth, appearing as if they had been badly eaten and discolored by some corrosive agent.' "

"And that's supposed to be healthy?"

"Of course not, Larry. Discoloration of the teeth only happens when we take in too much fluoride. But when we get the right amount, tooth enamel gets harder, so we have fewer cavities."

"True, fluoride does create an initial hardening of tooth enamel and resistance to decay, but that effect only lasts one year. *One year, Carter.* Then, if excessive fluoride consumption is continued, the teeth will mottle and discolor.

Your scientists call this 'dental fluorosis.' If fluoride consumption continues, teeth may become brittle and eventually it may become impossible for them to hold ordinary fillings. And when decay does set in, it's disastrous. Fillings won't work, and caps or crowns are necessary to preserve the tooth."

"Larry, you asked me how fluoridation got started."

"Yes. Continue, Carter. This has got to be good."

"In 1938, Gerald H. Cox, a biochemist with the Mellon Institute, came up with the idea of fluoridating drinking water supplies."

"And he got this idea all by himself?"

"He was supported by an attorney named Oscar Ewing."

"What did these two have in common, Carter?"

"Both had been associated with the Aluminum Company of America."

"Ah ha!" he exclaimed in triumph. "Do you suppose the fact that fluoride is a waste byproduct of aluminum manufacture had anything to do with their decision to dump fluoride into your drinking water, Carter?"

"Don't be ridiculous, Larry. Men don't work that way."

"Don't be too sure, Carter. Ewing, a former counsel of ALCOA, later became director of the Social Security of the U.S. Public Health Service. He played a very important part in persuading that organization to endorse fluoridation."

"Maybe. Ewing was just a lawyer, but Cox was a biochemist, Larry. He knew what he was doing."

"But nobody else did, Carter. Without any scientific studies, fluoridation experiments on humans began in 1945. Oh, excuse me. I shouldn't say 'experiments.' They called them 'demonstrations.' "

"How else could we find out if fluoridation works against dental decay, Larry?" I asked reasonably. "One fluoridation demonstration began in Grand Rapids, Michigan, using Muskegon, Michigan as the non-fluoridated control city. Another commenced in Newburgh, New York, and Kingston acted as the control area."

"Carter, it's inconceivable that the New York State Department of Health would consider subjecting 40,000 innocent humans to even a minute amount of one of the most toxic substances known to mankind without ever having done animal studies to prove its safety. There were no proper dental examinations with x-rays; no provision for the study of the possible effects of fluoride on adults; and no provisions for double-blind control measures, which are normally set up in medical trials of a substance."

"Look, Larry, I remember the Grand Rapids study. It was reported on television and in newspapers and magazines that cavities were reduced there because of the fluoridation program."

"Yes, I know. I remember also. The Grand Rapids-Muskegon study is often cited in support of artificially fluoridating city water. But, here's what *really* happened. Five years into what was supposed to be a ten-year study, fluoride advocates found that the decay rate of non-fluoridated Muskegon was decreasing at the same rate as fluoridated Grand Rapids. Because this data didn't support fluoride, Muskegon was dropped from the study as the control city. The published report states only that tooth decay dropped in Grand Rapids, inferring that fluoride caused the decrease.

"If you will remember, Carter, the Newburgh and Grand Rapids trials were supposed to continue for a full ten years. But, thanks to some spectacular publicity, you humans were ready to be convinced that fluoridation was a good thing. Humans weren't willing to wait. Cities all over the U.S. began fluoridating their water supplies in the belief that their children wouldn't have to go to the dentist so often."

"I don't care what you say, Larry. Scientists are usually in science for the love of it, and only rarely for hope of personal financial gain. Any corruption is more likely to be of an elusive intellectual kind, rather than overtly financial, as you seem to be implying."

"However, Carter, it is possible that the scientific community as a whole may be the victim of outside commercial pressures and scientific truth gets sidetracked. That's quite another matter."

"What commercial pressures are you talking about?"

"Don't you remember discovering that there is a direct commercial interest in promoting fluoridation through various grants and subsidies, Carter? For example, the Sugar Research Foundation is vitally interested in any research which appears to show that tooth decay can be effectively controlled without restricting the intake of sugar. The American Water Works Association enthusiastically endorsed fluoridation, but they are largely sustained by chemical and aluminum companies, the same companies which either sell or manufacture fluoride as a byproduct of their main industries."

"What you're suggesting is very hard for me to believe, Larry."

"Oh, really? Maybe this will convince you. The Aluminum Company of Canada actually published a full-page advertisement promoting 'Alcan Sodium Fluoride.' And for many years, the American Medical Association derived a large portion of the income for its annual budget from advertisers of drugs. Because they are beholden to the drug producers for so much of their income, your AMA is held captive by pharmaceutical interests.

"Another thing, Carter. Fluoride can't actually penetrate teeth, because both carry a negative charge. To overcome this, it would be necessary to reverse the negative charge of tooth enamel by introducing a fluoride salt into saliva and then passing an electric current through the mouth when you brush your teeth, thereby turning your mouth into a kind of organic battery."

"That would be dangerous, Wouldn't it, Larry?"

"You would certainly experience some physical discomfort,"

he said sarcastically. "Your head would ache and teeth holding fillings would be painful."

"So, if fluoride can't actually penetrate the teeth, then brushing with it doesn't help reduce cavities. Right?"

"Brushing helps remove bacteria, Carter. But fluoride is a poison."

"I've been brushing my teeth with fluorided toothpaste for many years, Larry. Obviously, I'm still alive."

"Thanks to me, Carter, and many of my colleagues who gave up their lives for you."

"Come on, Larry." I was skeptical. "Fluoride really can't be all that bad."

"I know how bad it is, Carter. The question is, does it really do any good?"

"Okay, Larry. The bottom line. Does fluoride prevent cavities?"

"No. Studies by the U.S. Public Health Service show no difference in tooth decay rates between high and low fluoridated areas. British, Danish, and Japanese studies all agree that fluoride does not reduce the incidence of tooth decay."

I was searching for some shred of logic in support of fluoridation. "Is fluoride an important nutrient then?"

"Fluoride is not an essential nutrient. It is a documented fact that as little as one-tenth of an ounce of fluoride can cause death. When sold over-the-counter, fluoride comes in a can marked with the universal symbol of poison, the skull and cross bones."

"Still Larry, all over the country, fluoride is routinely added to city water supplies as a dental decay preventive."

"What do I have to do to get through to you, human? The optimal fluoride is advertised to be 1 part-per-million. We know that the ingestion of drinking water containing as little as 1.2 to 3 ppm of fluorine will cause such developmental disturbances in bones as osteosclerosis, spondilitis, and osteoporosis and goiters as well."

"Larry, the World Health Organization endorses fluoridation."

"The World Health Organization voted on fluoridation when only 60 out of 1,000 delegates were present. It was no accident that these 60 delegates happened to be the few who were in favor of fluoride. Even so, the resolution was passed with the recommendation that more studies be done on the fluoride content of diets, the effects of fluoride on the human body, and the effects of excessive intake from various sources."

"There, you see. They're trying."

"But they directly contradicted themselves, Carter. Only a year later, the WHO press officer warmly recommended fluoridation and pronounced it 'absolutely safe.' "

I was beginning to feel that I was clutching at straws. "Maybe they found something in that year that enabled them to make that statement, Larry."

"I have checked the bone structure of your cranium, Carter. It doesn't appear to be as thick as you seem to be right now. You don't want to recognize that a gigantic power structure is pushing fluoridation. The Public Health Service spends hundreds of millions of dollars every year on grants, cooperative programs, and salary supplements, all to support fluoride. By these means, they have welded state and county organizations into one completely docile and responsive body amenable to the slightest pressure from Washington. Endorsements from the national organizations are solicited by a number of the same humans. In most instances, these same humans act unilaterally and function simultaneously in all of the various organizations."

He continued his lecture. "Public health officials endorse fluoridation, but then they put on another of their hats, call themselves a state organization, and endorse it all over again. The World Health Organization is financed by the U.S. Public Health Service. It's no surprise to find that they endorse flouridation. The power apparatus spends millions every year in an effort to force water works to accept their recommendations. They have dozens of public relations experts. Every state organization has at least one. All are industriously engaged in putting out prepared stories endorsing fluoride. No schools, colleges, or even independent medical research institutions dare criticize fluoride because they receive public health grants. By the same token, no big food, beverage, or drug company will speak critically about fluoride because they are under the supervision of your Food & Drug Administration, and the FDA is a branch of the Public Health Service."

"Motive. Larry, there has to be a motive. What is it?"

"You want a motive, Carter? I'll give you 'motive.' What would you do if you produced over half a million tons of poison every year that you had to get rid of? That seems to be motive enough. Statistics from the National Society of Sciences show that U.S. industries pump over 100,000 tons of fluoride into the atmosphere every year, and dispose of another 500,000 tons by dumping it into your drinking water."

"Fluoride is a poisonous waste?"

He exploded. "Yes! What do you think I've been telling you, Carter? Fluoride is an industrial waste product occurring in the manufacture of aluminum. And, yes, it is this same industrial waste that your health officials use to fluoridate your drinking water.

"All right, Carter, I can see you're having trouble grasping this. Admittedly, fluoride is a difficult pill to swallow, in more ways than one. Maybe this story will help:

"Mason City, Iowa was the scene of an interesting fluoridation campaign. The fluoride drum-beaters descended on Mason City with their usual misleading literature. The hometown paper was persuaded to join the crusade. Endorsements by so-called experts were introduced, and civic groups joined the parade. Local doctors issued statements about the deplorable state of Mason City kid's teeth. They made it look as if the decay rate was so appalling that local dentists couldn't handle the terrible situation. A Dr. Henshaw, an employee of the Iowa State Department of Health, came to town to display his charts and graphs which ostensibly showed that adding 1 ppm fluoride to the drinking water would lower the incidence of dental decay in Mason City children by 65 percent.

"But Mason City was in for a big surprise. Some forward-thinking scientists tested the existing Mason City water supply and found that it already contained 1.25 ppm of naturally-occurring fluoride, even more than the 'magic' amount that the experts claimed was needed to cut the decay rate."

I laughed out loud. "The fluoride fanciers probably felt very foolish, Larry. That's a great story. Do you have any more?"

"You bet, but they aren't funny. I've been saving them up to put in this book. Did you know that scientists at the Seibersdorf Research Center in Austria have reported that as little as 1 ppm of fluoride slows down the activity of the immune system?"

"I'll bet you've been waiting a long time to get in that bit of information," I commented.

He ignored me. "And did you know that fluoride can cause various genetic and chromosomal damage in plants, animals, and humans?"

"That would make them mutant cells; possible cancer cell candidates," I answered slowly. Fluoride was fast becoming a horror story.

"Right. Using bone marrow and testes cells, a U.S. geneticist has demonstrated that the degree of chromosomal damage increases proportionally in direct relation to the amount of fluoride in water. You must realize, Carter, that the soldiers of your immune defense forces are slowed down every time you drink fluoridated and polluted water. We have to search out and destroy all the damaged cells in your entire body.

These harmful substances that we have to defend against increase the possibility that you will develop cancer. When we're chasing them down, we can't be taking care of precancerous cells, the mutants.

"There's more, Carter. Using the same level of fluoride commonly put into U.S. drinking water, scientists at the Nippon Dental College of Japan have determined that even this minute amount of fluoride is capable of transforming normal cells into cancer cells. At a meeting of the Japanese Association of Cancer Research in Osaka in 1982, the researchers reported: 'Last year at this meeting, we showed that sodium fluoride, which is being used for the prevention of dental caries, induces chromosomal aberrations in the irregular synthesis of DNA. This year, we report findings that show malignant transformation of cells is induced by sodium fluoride.' "

"I can't believe it, Larry! That's amazing. How about similar studies in the U.S.?"

"As incredible as it may seem, Carter, research by the American Cancer Institute conducted as far back as 1963 clearly shows that even very low levels of fluoride increase the incidence of melanotic tumors in experimental laboratory animals by a frightening 12 to 100 percent. I can tell you that similar types of transformations have been observed in humans.

"It's not as if your human experts don't know, Carter. For example, Dean Burk, chief chemist emeritus of the NCI has been quoted as saying, 'In point of fact, fluoride causes more human cancer death and causes it faster than any other chemical.'

"Further, the U.S. Center for Disease Control has confirmed an increased cancer death rate in humans living in fluoridated communities, particularly among persons 45 and older. The findings of John Yiamouyiannis, Ph.D., president of the Safe Water Foundation in Columbus, Ohio and Dr. Dean Burk of the NCI agree with those of the Center for Disease Control. These scientists have documented what they say is a 10 percent fluoride-related increase in the death rate in cities supplying fluoridated water."

"You're scaring me, Larry. What you're saying is that no amount of fluoride ingestion is really safe."

"Data from the U.S. Center for Disease Control shows that deaths from all causes are at least 5 percent higher in fluoridated areas, Carter. All by itself, fluoride is deadly. Think what we have to contend with when it's combined with all the other pollutants in the water you drink every day.

"Here's another story for you, Carter. There's a little town in Turkey known as 'the village where people age before their time.' Turkish scientists have discovered that every single inhabitant suffers from a bone disease."

"I'm afraid to ask. Do they know why, Larry?"

"The village well is polluted with fluoride."

"Sad."

"If you think that's sad, Carter, you should know that all over the world parents are discovering the dangers of fluoride to their sorrow. A little 18-month old Australian youngster died from fluoride poisioning after he ate 4 fluoride tablets. In New York, a 3-year old human died after having his teeth treated with fluoride as a decay preventive. The dental hygienist forgot to tell the youngster to rinse and spit. He drank a cup of water and ingested a lethal dose of the poison. Yet another U.S. dental hygienist witnessed the death of a tiny human after fluoride treatment. The child went into convulsions and died in the dental chair. The parents never knew the truth. The child's death certificate says he died of a heart attack."

"All right, Larry. I don't want to hear any more."

"These are all reports I picked up while you were reading the newspaper over the years, Carter."

"I don't remember, I guess."

"They didn't mean anything to you at the time, Carter. Do you remember the 'Annapolis' story?"

"No."

"In 1979, up to 50 ppm of fluoride was accidentally pumped into the city water supplies in Annapolis, Maryland. An estimated 10,000 humans exhibited acute symptoms of fluoride poisoning, Carter. And about 50,000 ingested a poisonous concentration of this lethal substance. Over five times as many humans died of heart attacks during the week following the malfunction. The citizens were not told of the spill when it occurred and couldn't take steps to protect themselves."

"That's awful, Larry. Why weren't they told?"

"When the story became known and the city fathers were called to task, a public health official said, "We didn't want to jeopardize the fluoridation program.' I ask you, Carter, if the officials of one state admit to having covered-up the problem, where else has it happened? Maybe malfunctioning equipment dumps excessive amounts of fluoride into the drinking water without the public ever knowing about it. As a matter of fact, fluoride spills are on record as having occurred in Pennsylvania, North Carolina, California, Maine, New Mexico, and Michigan, as well as in Maryland."

"Okay, Larry. No more. You've made your point. Water is vital, but it must be clean water."

"Pure water."

"And where do you suppose I can get pure water?"

"From the fresh whole foods you eat. You see, the cells of plants need pure water, too. This water becomes the juice or nectar as it's filtered through the roots, trunk, and stems of the plants."

I agreed readily. "That's a good idea. Apple juice, orange juice, and tomato juice all taste great, and they're good for you and me, too."

"However, Carter, I must point out that most of your fruit juices are concentrated, meaning that you have to add water to reconstitute them."

"Is there anything wrong with that?"

"Not if you're getting your water from a pure source."

"Oh, of course. It wouldn't do any good to drink juice if I add water straight from the tap."

"You'll just have to figure out how to remove the impurities so that the only ingredients in your water are two-parts hydrogen and one-part oxygen. Nothing else."

"I'll work on it and get back to you, buddy."

"Don't drag your feet, Carter," he said smartly. "Remember, fluoride is a cumulative poison, and you've been using fluoridated water for a long time now."

With Larry's injunction to 'hurry' ringing in my eyes, I mounted an intensive investigation over the next few days. I talked to everyone I could find with any degree of expertise on the subject of water. I investigated the companies who deliver big jugs of bottled water to homes and found that some provided 'purified' water 'purified' with chemicals, while some maintain their own wells. Remembering what Larry had said, I wasn't sure of the purity of groundwater wells. I read the labels on all the bottled waters in the supermarket. Some sounded OK to me, but none offered Larry's 'recipe' of two-parts hydrogen and one-part oxygen. Besides, it's a nuisance to carry home bottled water all the time. I finally came to the conclusion that my solution to water pollution had to be a home purifying system that I could hook up to my kitchen faucet, so I began looking into various systems. All the literature was expertly prepared and the claims made were many.

But I wasn't completely satisfied until I found the *Clear-Energy Purification/Oxygenation System*. This company has documentation showing that the Purewater system will remove both fluoride and chlorine, along with all the peripheral pollutants and groundwater contaminates that abound everywhere. For my money, reverse osmosis coupled with proper activated charcoal filters qualified as the best home water purification process available. Research developed through the U.S. Department of the Interior says, "Reverse osmosis is highly effective at removing pollutants from water."

How does this marvelous system work? The process works a bit like the kidney dialysis machine, in that it employs the use of a semi-permeable membrane. After the charcoal prefilters have removed most of the organic chemicals, bacteria and other larger contaminants, the water pressure forces the contaminated tap water into direct contact with a specially designed semipermeable membrane. Tiny little molecules of sparkling pure water and molecules of pure oxygen pass easily through the membrane. But chemicals (including chlorine and fluoride), contaminants, pollutants, and gunk are screened out and flushed down the drain into the sewer where they belong. The *ClearEnergy System* delivers only the highest-quality crystal-clear pure water and pure oxygen, nothing else.

Another thing I like about this company is that they offer two different sizes (and prices) for home use. The ClearEnergy is available in a counter-top model and an under-sink model. (either model may easily be taken with you if you move) In other words, there's a ClearEnergy unit available for the apartment, home or office that will fit comfortably into almost every budget. The carbon prefilters are designed to last from three to five years with trouble-free service and the system has electronic and pressure devices for monitoring the purity of the water.

And, yes, Larry approves, so I'm sure he would want me to tell the reader where this wonderful system can be found.

There might be a distributor in your area for ClearEnergy Systems, but if not, you may contact the following:

New Dimensions Distributors
16548 E. Laser Drive, #A-7
Fountain Hills, Arizona 85268
Call: 1-800-624-7114 Toll-Free Nationwide
In Arizona (602), Call: 1-837-8322

Bibliography

Alabaster, MD, O: What You Can Do To Prevent Cancer. New York: Simon and Schuster, 1985.

Bragg, ND, PhD, PC: The Shocking Truth About Water. Santa Barbara, CA: Health Science.

Chen,PS: Inorganic, Organic and Biological Chemistry. New York: Harper and Rowe, 1979.

Gotzsche, AL: The Fluoride Question. Briercliff Manor, New York: Stein and Day, 1975.

Guyton, AC: Text Book of Medical Physiology. Philadelphia: WB Saunders Co, 1986.

Salsbury, KH and Johnson, EL: Indispensable Cancer Hand-book, New York: Seaview Books, 1981.

Yiamouyiannis, PhD, John: Fluoride: The Aging Factor. Delaware, Ohio: Health Action Press, 1983.

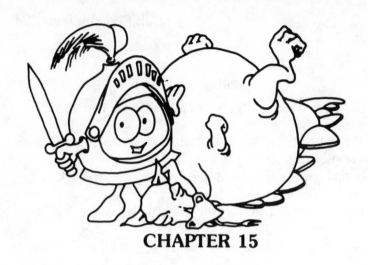

CHAPTER 15

CELLULAR COMMUNICATION

I was seated at my word processor musing on the universal importance of communication and wondering what put that particular subject in my head. Because I'm a writer, I just naturally like to put words on paper. I looked at the screen and saw that I had written:

The ability to read and write should never be taken for granted. Scholars from every manifestation have only been able to record the wisdom of the ages by writing down their insights and storing them in some form, whether in books or on stone tablets or papyrus scrolls. Many of the greatest thinkers of history have long since passed on, but they have left us a priceless legacy of timeless writings. We are truly blessed to be able to tell each other our innermost thoughts. Communication is certainly one of the greatest blessings a benevolent Creator ever bestowed upon us.

Larry's familiar voice buzzed in my left ear. "I couldn't agree with you more, Carter. Life simply could not exist without the God-given ability to communicate."

"Oh, hi, Larry. It's getting so that I don't know what I'm going to write when I sit down at my computer. I guess you really appreciate our ability to communicate. We've both been taking advantage of our oldest method of communication-storage lately, our libraries, and the very latest, our computers."

"You've come a long way in the last thousand years as a super-intelligent species, Carter. But you don't have the corner on intelligence-gathering, storage, or communication."

"Wait a minute, Larry. The ability to communicate intelligently is what sets man apart from all other animals. That, and our unique opposable thumb."

"Sometimes you amaze me, Carter. For a species which claims to have a superior intelligence, you humans sure seem to have your heads in the sand. All animals of every kingdom have the ability to communicate in their own way."

"Oh, I know that, Larry. Dogs bark at the moon and cats meow on the back fence. But you really can't call that communication."

"Are you trying to tell me that some of the noises you make are any better?" he asked derisively.

"What do you mean?"

"Explain to me how humans use the sounds of music as a method of communication."

"That's easy, Larry. Music communicates mood, sends various messages, signals ethnic background, culture, attitudes, and even dreams."

"Right. Therefore, communication doesn't necessarily have to be in spoken or written words."

"Of course not," I agreed readily. "We use signs and symbols and even a series of lights to get across the vital signals needed by modern transportation systems so that we won't run into each other."

"When a wild dog places his paws on the back of another dog to show his position as a superior in the pecking order, would that qualify as a form of communication?"

"I guess so."

"Whales, the largest living animal on this earth, sing to each other. Their songs are so complex that your scientists listen to them in amazement."

"I know. That's partly because whales seem to have their songs memorized. They are able to produce the same song-sounds years apart."

"Would you call that a form of communication, Carter?"

"Yes."

"What do they say?"

"I don't know, Larry," I answered in exasperation. "Even our scientists don't know. How can you expect *me* to know when our greatest scientists are still confused?"

"I don't, Carter. I just expect you to accept the fact that humans aren't the only creatures with the ability to communicate."

"Oh, Larry, we've been talking to other animals for ages. German Shepherds and Collie dogs have been helping the shepherds of the field herd sheep and cattle for centuries. With just a hint of what the shepherd requires his dogs to do, the dogs go forth and do it, as long as it's something a dog can handle.

"Today, Larry, dogs are both pets and guard dogs," I continued. "But to live in this modern society with so many people, they have had to learn a whole new set of commands, like 'heel,' and 'lie down,' and how to communicate when they want to go outside, and when not to bark."

"Yes. Pets have to put up with an awful lot to live with humans."

"They're smart, too. We've been using dogs in circus shows for ages, because they're able to understand what we want."

"Have you ever asked a dog what it wants, Carter?"

"Don't be silly, Larry. A dog just wags its tail, pants when it's hot, barks for whatever reason, and scratches at the door."

"Maybe you should listen the next time."

"We would listen, if dogs had anything to say," I said reasonably. "We haven't been very successful in teaching dogs to talk, but birds are another story. We've been able to teach them to say all sorts of things, like 'polly wants a cracker,' for instance. I have a parakeet that makes all sorts of sounds, almost as if it's carrying on an involved conversation. But we can't pick out any words in all the garble.

"We've even been able to talk to plants, Larry. A group of 7th graders planted mung beans in small individual pots, using the same soil and plant-food in each and exposing them all to the same amount of sun and water. But they talked and sang to half of them. The mung beans that received the extra attention grew twice as fast as those who received only physical care."

"That's great, Carter," he enthused. "What did the plants say?"

"Plants don't talk, Larry," I said patiently.

"Don't be too sure. I remember your watching an experiment conducted by scientists during which they connected a plant up to a volt meter so that they could measure minute electrical impulses."

"Oh, yes. That was on television. If I remember correctly, one of the scientists killed a mouse in the presence of the plant and the plant registered a measurable increase in electrical energy transmitted."

"Right, Carter. Do you remember what happened next?"

"Sure, Every time the scientist who had killed the mouse walked into the same room with the wired-up plant, the plant registered 'fear' by putting out increased electrical impulses."

"Now, tell me this, Carter: Was the scientist communicating with that plant?"

"Yes. By scaring the poor thing."

"Did the plant communicate with the scientist?"

"By displaying fear, it sure did." I saw where he was heading. "Larry, this conversation is getting ridiculous."

"You might think so. I don't."

"I refuse to go outside and apologize to my grass because

I have to mow it. Also, I happen to enjoy playing a game of golf now and again. I can hear me now: 'Oops, sorry, dear divot. I didn't mean to tear you away from your neighborhood.'

"Carter, as a species, you humans have been extremely inconsiderate of all the other wonders of God's creation. In fact, you haven't even been all that considerate of your own kind. You humans make war on each other and murder each other. You have polluted your environment and rendered your waters unfit for consumption. You humans are certainly not very considerate of my world."

I was getting angry. "Now just a minute, Larry, I've made a lot of changes in my lifestyle for you."

"Stop taking everything so personally, Carter. I'm talking about the whole human race in general. You are doing better but you still live in a polluted environment that humans have contaminated."

I was a bit mollified. "Okay, I see your point. What do you want us to do about it?"

"First, give the rest of God's creatures credit for the amount of intelligence they possess."

"Can you be a bit more specific?"

"Have you heard of 'Alex the Parrot?' "

"I've seen many parrots, but I don't recall being introduced to one named Alex."

"That's all right, Carter. Very few humans have. Ever since Irene Pepperberg, an ethologist at Northwestern University, bought Alex at a pet store nine years ago, he has been demonstrating abilities that most scientists believe belong to the realm of man."

"Like what?"

"Alex labels objects. He perceives quantities. He requests specific foods. And he also generalizes concepts, like colors and shapes, and applies them to things he's never seen before. In short, Alex doesn't mimic. He communicates."

"Alex is a rare bird indeed," I observed.

"Not really, Carter. Irene Pepperberg took the time not only to teach Alex, but also to listen to him. Other parrots can do the same things."

"I guess you're right, Larry. I've read about a pygmy chimpanzee who understands dozens of words, and another chimp in Reno, Nevada who was taught sign language, the hand-language of the deaf. This chimp was eventually able to master over 170 words."

"Carter, dolphins and sea lions have progressed even further. Some grasp not only words, but some basic rules of grammar."

"I'm convinced, Larry. I guess animals have much more complex communications skills than we ever imagined."

"Why stop at the animals? How about all living things? One of your problems is that you humans believe that all other life forms should learn your language. You humans seem to think your spoken and written methods of communication are the only forms of communication in the world. Have you ever thought that maybe it isn't the inability of other creatures to communicate that stands in the way, but your refusal to accept the possibility that other beings have methods of communication just as complex and complete as yours?"

He continued, "You humans expect dolphins, parrots, and chimps to think and communicate the same way you do. If you really want to communicate with other life forms, why don't you try to think like they do? If you want to communicate with the cells of your body, you're going to have to learn to think as we do. Why don't you humans try learning *our* language, instead of expecting us to learn yours? Carter, if you went to Japan to live, wouldn't you learn to speak Japanese?"

"Yes, I would, Larry," I answered apologetically. "I can see I've been handling this all wrong. You're the one who made an effort to communicate with me. I am now ready to learn how you communicate."

"Carter, what did you just do?"

"What? When?"

"With your hands."

"I'm typing."

"Besides that."

"Oh. I scratched my nose."

"Why?"

"Because it itched, of course."

"But you didn't first 'think' about scratching. Did you?"

"No. It was an automatic reflex, I guess."

"And did you know that millions of cells were involved with that little activity? All the cells involved received their own set of instructions even faster than your ability to think 'scratch.' "

"Sure, " I answered agreeably. "The muscle cells of my biceps had to move my forearm. My hand had to rotate to position my fingers. My fingers had to move to my nose and then move back and forth on the surface of my skin with just the right degree of pressure needed to relieve the itch, but without causing any damage."

"How did you know how much pressure to apply, or when you had scratched the itch sufficiently?"

"I guess I had to depend on the nerve cells of the surface of my nose and fingertips to tell the other nerve cells of the muscles of my arm, hand, and fingers how fast to move and when to stop." Simply scratching an itch was more complicated than I had ever dreamed.

"Carter, can you imagine what would happen if all your cellular communication systems broke down, even just for a moment?"

"I never thought about it," I acknowledged. "What would happen?" Suddenly I jumped and hollered "Ouch!"

"That's a verbal reactionary exclamatory response to an immediate awareness of neural transmitters sending messages of early warnings of impending serious injury to large numbers of cells."

"What happened, Larry? I tried to scratch my nose again,

and ended up slapping myself in the face and poking myself in the eye. Did you have something to do with that?" I asked suspiciously.

"That's just a demonstration of what can happen when your cellular communications break down for a mere moment, Carter."

My feelings were hurt and my eye was tearing madly. "You didn't have to do that, Larry. We have examples of neural miscommunication in Alzheimer's Disease, cerebral palsy, and epilepsy."

"That demonstration was only to point out to you, Carter, that cellular communication is far more sophisticated than the means of communication that you humans rely on. For example, your immediate response to a slap on the face and poke in the eye was 'ouch.' It was an immediate reaction. You didn't need time to think it over. Right?"

"Well, yes."

"The split second after the collision between your hand and face and your finger and your eye, the cells of the muscles of your eyelid, lips, tongue, chest, and diaphragm all received their own definite and very well-coordinated instructions on how to react to the emergency. We cells couldn't function effectively if we had to put our messages into the extremely slow method of communication you call 'thinking.' And trying to 'talk' to one another would be even worse."

I laughed. "And I guess it would take literally an entire lifetime of some cells if you had to send a neural message by writing a letter."

"You got that right, Carter! To us cells, it would be more like an eternity."

"If even thinking is too slow, how do you suggest humans communicate with our cells then?"

"You pray to your Creator, don't you, Carter?"

"Yes. You've been with me long enough to know that I pray many times throughout the day."

"Why?"

"Because humans have been told to pray by our prophets and so instructed in our holy writings."

"And who is listening?"

"I suppose God and His angels."

"Anyone else?"

"You?"

"We have that capability. When you ask for health and strength, you feel good about your relationship with your Creator and your fellow beings. We receive the very strong message that everything is just great with you. We cells all share in a great sense of accomplishment. A human might express well-being and satisfaction with his life by saying 'Everything is copasetic.' We say to ourselves, ' Everything is homeostatic.' "

"Wow!" I was impressed. 'So my prayers go in both directions. This could explain miracles, or faith healings, or . . ."

"Not so fast," he interrupted. "A little knowledge can get you into trouble fast. Keep in mind, your Creator is my Creator also. Your holy writ declares that you 'are made in His image,' and that you are. But that also means we are made in the image of His cells."

I was stunned at the thought. "That's heavy."

"But logical, Carter. To achieve your eternal goals, humans are required to be like Him. So also, for us cells to be successful in our own realm, we have to obey the physical laws of the body. There are physical laws irrevocably decreed and recorded in the DNA upon which your health is predicated. When you receive the blessing of good health, it is by obedience to those laws upon which health is predicated. Your good health is not accidental. I don't want to toot my own horn, Carter, but it takes a lot of hard work on our part to keep you healthy."

I was still stuck on his earlier statement and struggling to understand. "So cellular communication can come in the form of prayers, hopes, dreams, visualization, and even direct verbal commands? Is that right, Larry?"

"I guess you can say that," he responded.

"Someone else has said it much better, Larry. 'As a man thinketh in his heart, so he is.' "

"That saying should be 'As a man thinketh in his cells, so he is.' Because we cells are so aware of the way you humans regard yourselves, many of the illnesses man experiences you bring on yourselves by your 'stinkin thinkin.' "

I laughed at his phrasing. "What do you mean, Larry?"

"Worry, fear, anger, anxiety, and guilt are examples of feelings that only humans experience, Carter. All this 'stinkin thinkin' causes your hormone-producing glands to send destructive messages to your cells. We listen and obey. Some cells begin to produce chemical messages of doom and destruction, which are transmitted to other cells of the body. These messages are misinterpreted by the rest of the cells. In turn, they respond by misfunctioning. A chemical imbalance can show up as hives, allergies, rashes, or twitches. Sometimes you humans call it 'stress' and let it go at that. At other times, symptoms of a chemical imbalance can mimic an illness and are classified and treated as such."

"These must be the psychosomatic illnesses I've heard about."

"Yes. And sometimes they're harder to deal with than a physical condition, because there's no real enemy to attack and vanquish, just a miscommunication. You humans try to solve the problem by taking something foreign into the body in an effort to relieve your symptoms, but that just masks the real problem. Then we cells have to try to eliminate the foreign particles in the drugs you're taking, and we have to put up with unacceptable living conditions while we're trying to do our duty."

I was a bit amused at his earnestness. "Larry, I don't know of any medical authority who would tell a patient that the reason he feels so lousy is because he hasn't taken his cells into his confidence."

"Get serious, Carter. Can you imagine what would happen if a doctor advised his patient to do that?"

"Sure. They'd send him to the funny farm."

"Ignorance! Stupid ignorance!! And this is what we have to contend with all the time."

"I'm sorry, Larry," I said gently, trying to defuse his anger. "I'm sure the AMA wouldn't put up with such a wide deviation from the conventional way of handling illness. We've always been led to believe that cells are deaf, dumb, and blind and incapable of communicating."

"Dumb', are we, Carter? Show me a scientist who can build a bone. Or one who can produce a red blood cell. Show me anyone who can construct the right kind of protein for the hair on your head. Better yet, show me a scientist who can isolate a single mutant cell, and then destroy it without injuring the surrounding cells.

"Oh, no, Carter. It's not we cells who are dumb. We were communicating with each other intimately within your body long before you went to school to learn your alphabet. Even before your best scientist was born, we built his body in accordance with the rigid blueprints contained in his DNA."

I had never heard him so angry. "I know, Larry. I know. You've proven to me that you know what life is all about," I answered in what I hoped was a soothing manner.

"No, Carter. I don't know everything about life. But I do know my job and how to do it," he snapped. "And from what I've learned about your means of communicating, I can safely say that your most sophisticated methods are archaic when compared to ours. As I see it, the problem is that you humans simply don't know our language. The sad part is that most of you refuse to acknowledge the possibility that other forms of intelligent life exist. You humans are too busy looking to the stars and searching for alien worlds from outer space, when you should be trying to communicate with your *inner space*.

"Listen, Carter, all the cells of your body have been talking back and forth in our own way since you were conceived. And we'll continue to communicate with each other until you die."

"And how do you recommend that humans learn how to communicate with cells, Larry?" I was getting a little testy myself.

"Haven't you been paying attention, Carter? That seems to be your main problem. Humans have been communicating their innermost thoughts to cells since mankind began. Many times, your prayers for health and peace of mind, wisdom, or physical fitness have been answered by us cells."

He was on shaky ground with me now. "Are you trying to tell me that you cells are playing God?"

"Sometimes I wonder about your intelligence, Carter. No, we don't presume to 'play God,' as you put it. But He created us to do our jobs. We do them. You receive the blessings of health. What's good for you is also good for us.

"And another method of cellular communication that you're not aware of, Carter, is dreaming. We use your sleeping time to organize your experiences and file them away in your cellular library. In this way, when it becomes necessary for you to remember and recall something, it's easy for us to know where to put our hands on it and we retrieve it instantly."

"That's a bit like the Dewey Decimal system libraries use for filing books, right?"

"Pish and tush, Carter." He dismissed the idea. "Don't compare that slow method of filing and retrieval to our lightning-fast sytem. Whatever you input just before you fall asleep becomes vitally important to us while you are sleeping. Many times, if you have a problem you find difficult to solve, just concentrate on it before you go to sleep. You'll awaken to find the solution ready and waiting. We use all your sleeping hours to logically come up with the ideal way to handle the problem. How's *that* for cellular communication?" he asked proudly.

"Great! Where were you when I was in school and

needed you?"

"How do you think you got those good grades on all the tests you crammed for?" he shot back. "We were right there with you. And that leads us into another area of cellular communication, Carter. Your formal education program. Every time you learn something, anything at all, it is indelibly recorded in the DNA of all the cells charged with the responsibility of reconstruction when called upon. Whether it is the cells of your muscles and the nerves of your fingertips as you type, or the big muscles of your legs as you run and jump, we learn as you learn."

"So you were in school learning right along with me," I mused.

"There's a difference between cells and humans, Carter. When you left school, your formal education stopped. We never stop. We're hungry for knowledge. We cells are learning all the time. Sometimes we learn the wrong things. When that happens, we become confused between the things we instinctively know are right for you, and the things you've been teaching us by following harmful practices. This comes under the heading of 'stress.' And it's a dangerous situation when your cells are not acting in your best interests because you're sending us the wrong signals."

"Stress, huh? Okay, Larry, what's the most stressful learning experience cells can have?"

"When our human learns from a doctor that cancer has been detected in his body."

"Why should that be stressful to you cells, Larry? The official diagnosis can't be a surprise to you. Wouldn't you already know the cancer is there?"

"Certainly, And we're already working on the problem. We don't need to be told our jobs. But a human doctor feels it's important to tell his patient how much time he has to live."

"I can see where a diagnosis of cancer can put terrific stress on a human, Larry. It's pretty scary. After all, a lot of cancers are terminal. But how can it shock or stress cells?"

"By the time the diagnosis is made, Carter, we usually have the cancer under control. But when a patient is told they have, say, six months to live, this message runs through the body like a shot of adrenalin. When the cells of the body receive it, they simply prepare the body for death. They give up and quit fighting. The immune system slows down and becomes inefficient, giving the cancer an opportunity to take over."

"Wow! That's devastating."

"It is six months later, Carter," he said definitively.

"What can we humans do to combat this effect, Larry?"

" 'Ye shall know the truth, and the truth shall make you free.' " he quoted.

"I guess that well-known scripture has real meaning even at the cellular level," I said thoughtfully.

"Truth is truth, Carter. Try this one on for size: 'Be ye therefore perfect, even as your Father in Heaven is perfect.' Of course, we have to revise it slightly to make it fit my situation. 'Be ye therefore perfect, even as the cells of your Father in Heaven are perfect.' That's what we're after, isn't it?"

"I guess so. Yes."

"So, Carter, another way of communicating with the cells of your body is by your attitude. More important than almost any other single factor to your total cell environment is your attitude toward life. A positive winning attitude puts all the cells of your body on notice that perfection is expected in the functioning of your body. I'm sure you've heard of humans who have overcome all odds and performed seeming miracles because they refused to accept physical illness."

"Yes. Our scientists call that 'psycho-immunity' and it involves strong visualization. A cancer patient might imagine that his lymphocytes are white knights in shining armor, and his cancer is a dragon. Every day, he sends his white knights out to fight the dragon and eventually the knights triumph."

"We would have fought the 'dragon' anyway, Carter.

But, when the patient is thinking positive thoughts, he isn't poisoning his internal environment with negative messages. The feeling of winning the battle and influencing the outcome is very favorable to us cells. This message is communicated throughout the body. All cells feel they are part of a winning team and remember that what they do really matters. All the cells of the body will pull together with perfect confidence that all the other cells will do their part. Then 'the body fitly framed together groweth into a holy temple in the Lord.' "

"Gee, Larry, I can't decide if you sound more like a minister or a physical fitness coach. I didn't know that you had it in you... er, me."

"Is there a difference? Carter, the most important possession you have is your body. And, since it happens to be made in the image of God, it happens to be my most important possession also. I guess this is the proper place to say that you should be involved in an exercise program religiously."

"Cute, Larry." I laughed. "But I thought we were talking about cellular communication in this chapter, not exercise."

"At the cellular level, there's no difference between cell communication and cell exercise, Carter. Everytime you exercise, you are telling each of us cells to adjust to the demands exercise makes on your entire body. We listen. We obey. We really don't have a choice."

"And your preferred exercise is?"

"An exercise that provides cellular stimulation for every cell in your body equally."

"You're talking about rebound exercise again, Larry."

"You took the words right out of my mouth, Carter."

"You don't have a mouth."

"I've been talking to you for too long. I'm beginning to think like a human."

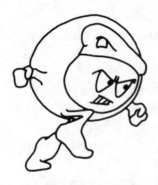

CHAPTER 16

SUPPLEMENTAL CELL FOOD

I yawned and stretched luxuriously as I mounted the Rebound for my wakeup workout. I was in mid-air when I heard Larry buzzing a 'good morning' in my right ear. We exchanged greetings of the day while I continued exercising to Larry's complete satisfaction. After I had gone through my favorite ten-minute bouncing routine on the Rebound, I made my way to the kitchen.

I took my bottle of Desert Gold bee pollen granules out of the refrigerator and dug into it with a spoon. As I savored the sweet-tart taste of the golden grains, I sipped a glass of freshly squeezed orange juice and spooned some low-fat cottage cheese into a small bowl, topping it off with a dollop of virgin C-Leinosan Linseed Oil. Since Larry had explained the importance of including the essential fatty acids in the diet to me, I had come to relish the rich distinctive taste of this ages-old natural dietary fat. I then fixed myself a bowl of whole-grain cereal and added a drizzle of raw honey and a sliced banana before I splashed on the low-fat milk.

"I approve, Carter," Larry said. "It's very gratifying to know that you've taken my teachings to heart."

"I really think I feel better since I've switched to cell-foods," I commented.

"I *know* you feel better, Carter," he shot back. "We cells don't have to work nearly as hard to keep your internal environment clean as we did before. We can really tell the difference now that you're drinking pure dechemicalized water and eating whole foods. By the way, we especially appreciate the boost we get from bee pollen."

"I do seem to remember reading that bee pollen helps the immune system, Larry, but I don't remember how it works."

"Do you remember the USDA report published by the National Cancer Institute back in 1948 concluding that bee pollen has a pronounced effect on malignant mammary tumors, Carter?"

"It must be buried in my memory banks somewhere, Larry, or you wouldn't know about it. But it seems to have escaped me. How about refreshing my memory?"

"Sure. Your U.S. scientists didn't pay much attention to this important study, Carter. William Robinson, M.D., of the U.S. Department of Agriculture proved that bee pollen added to food could prevent or slow down the development of cancerous mammary tumors in a special strain of mice bred to succumb to such tumors. In addition, existing tumors were reduced in size in the mice given bee pollen with their food."

"That's a pretty important finding, Larry."

"Scientists around the world agree, Carter. Dr. L.J. Hayes of the Apiculteur Haut-Chinois points out that bees sterilize the pollen they harvest with a secretion that helps us fight tumors. French researchers at the Institute of Bee Culture in Paris report that they have extracted the antibiotic factor present in the bee pollen and discovered that many harmful microbes are destroyed by bee pollen extract, including the sometimes deadly salmonella bacteria. That means we lymphos don't have to mess with them. Bee pollen is a mighty medicinal, Carter. It works effectively to normalize an organism that's out of sync and helps restore homeostasis. But it is as a mighty cell-food that we cells appreciate bee pollen most."

"Why is that, Larry?"

"Bee pollen is the most complete cell-food of all, Carter. Because it's the very essence of the flowering plant, each one of those tiny little grains contains a powerhouse of nutrients. Bee pollen provides us with all the important vitamins, minerals, enzymes, hormones, amino acids, carbohydrates, and trace elements we need to do our work, because the plant cells include all that in the pollen. We cells can only carry out our vital functions when we're well and truly nourished and working at top efficiency."

"That makes sense," I acknowledged. "I like the rather flowery taste of the raw granules myself, but some people don't. Is it okay to take a prepared bee pollen supplement instead?"

"It depends on how it's produced, Carter. Pure raw bee pollen granules are enzyme-active and all the nutrients nature intended are present. But if the bee pollen is subjected to too much heat in the processing, all the enzymes we need are destroyed. And if any kind of a supplement is junked up with a lot of unnecessary chemicals that we have to defend your body against, forget it. We'd really rather you ate the real thing."

"Since you gave me the responsibility of searching out the best sources of cell-foods, I've done a lot of homework, Larry, and. . ."

"I didn't *give* you that responsibility, Carter. It was yours all along," he said quickly.

"You're right, of course, Larry. But it was your teaching that made me realize how important cell food really is. It seems to me that the BioSan people do a really good job with all their products. I especially like their fresh *Desert Gold Bee Pollen Granules*. These pollen harvesters of domestic bee pollen exhibit a very high level of expertise in the development and production of all their products."

"Explain, Carter."

"My pleasure!" I said enthusiastically. "Desert Gold is harvested in the environmentally clean western states and is a complex blend of many different pollens. The fact that BioSan supplies a blend of bee pollens from many areas is important. Soil studies compiled by the U.S. Department of Agriculture show that there's no place left in the nation where the soil contains a complete complement of nutrients. Some areas are top-heavy in certain vital nutrients, and some are deficient in other nutrients."

"I see," Larry interjected. "When the nutrients aren't in the soil, they won't be present in plants grown in that soil, or in the pollen produced by the plants."

"Right. Being the smart little critters that they are, bees are programmed to collect superior pollens. BioSan remedies the deficiencies man has caused with his tinkering of the environment by blending the high-quality pollens harvested by the bees in many areas to insure that a complete complement of all nutrients is present in their Desert Gold bee pollen products."

"If that's Desert Gold bee pollen you've been taking, Carter, I can tell that they use a cold-processing procedure. The enzymes we cells need were certainly alive and active in that spoonful of bee pollen you ate this morning, and the nutrients and important trace elements were most welcome, too."

"I'm glad to hear you say that, little buddy. Another thing you'll like about the BioSan products is that they contain no artificial flavors, colors, sugars, starches, or unwanted chemical preservatives."

"That is good news, Carter. I have a confession to make. As long as a dietary supplement is produced with natural elements and doesn't contain a mess of manmade chemicals that we have to clean up and defend against, we cells can't tell whether you are eating a whole food or supplying us with the nutrients we need in supplement form."

"No kidding!"

" 'Kidding' is a human trait, Carter. You've known me long enough to know that I never 'kid,' " he said primly. "I say exactly what I mean. I mean exactly what I say."

I laughed aloud at his pomposity, and then decided I'd better apologize. "I'm sorry, Larry. I didn't mean to hurt your feelings," I said with a smile.

"I don't have 'feelings' either, Carter. But we're straying off the subject. What other good cell-foods have you discovered in supplement form?"

"I think you'll approve of the *Bee Pollesan* capsule formula, Larry. These caps are formulated with superior quality Desert Gold bee pollen and royal jelly, plus the herbs Gotu Kola and high-potency Siberian ginseng. As you already know, I like the pure Desert Gold granules, but my wife prefers the Bee Pollesan capsules."

"It sounds like the BioSan people have a bee pollen product to suit any human's tastes, Carter."

"They sure do. And I also discovered some very tasty highly-nutritious bee pollen 'candy' bars, made by The C C Pollen Company. My personal favorite is *The President's Lunch*. This is a delicious combination of natural things like oats, peanut butter, sunflower seeds, raisins, and honey. It's beefed up with 260 mg of quality bee pollen. The children like *The President's Choice* best. It's the same bar, but it contains twice as much bee pollen and is coated with carob, the natural chocolate."

"I guess I'll never understand why humans like to eat things that taste good, Carter. Cells don't care about things like that. We're only concerned with the nutrients you send us."

"I know that, Larry. But there's nothing wrong with nutrition that satisfies *our* craving for something sweet, as well as satisfying *your* need for cell food, is there?"

"Whatever gets you humans eating cell food is all right in my book, Carter. What about the other bars? You said there were five."

"Yes. Bonnie likes *The First Lady's Lunch* because it contains almonds and dates, instead of peanut butter and raisins. Peanut butter isn't one of her favorite foods. Every so often, especially when we're going out to dinner, Bonnie will skip lunch and munch a bar. At just 150 calories, this bar replaces a high calorie meal very effectively with good nutrition. *The First Lady's Choice* is the same bar with 520 mg of bee pollen, all richly swathed in carob. *The Executive Sweet* is a solid block of carob with a whopping 2080 mg of bee pollen blended right in. The company calls this one the answer to a chocoholic's prayer. It's very rich. In fact, any of these bars qualify as a good meal replacement in the form of a sweet treat. They're all enriched with the dynamite nutrition of quality bee pollen, too.

"There's still more, Larry. The C C Pollen Company also offers propolis and royal jelly. Do you have anything you want to say about these beehive products?"

"Certainly. The saps and resins of the trees and leafbuds that the bees combine with beeswax and use to manufacture propolis results in a biologically-active and effective medicinal compound that is also a highly beneficial form of preventive medicine."

"Yes. And that's why propolis is widely used by the medical profession abroad in special Apitherapy Clinics. Some of them call it 'Russian penicillin,' because it is the strongest natural antibiotic ever discovered and has been widely researched by USSR scientists. In medicine, propolis is prized for its antibacterial, antiviral, and antifungal properties, effective even against bacteria resistant to some of today's modern drugs, such as tetracycline and erythromycin."

"In addition," Larry broke in, "propolis will help reduce your susceptibility to colds, respiratory infections, sore throats, and flu, and it will dramatically help all your cells speed healing when taken regularly. Propolis is strong preventive medicine *and* a very effective natural remedy. If we stretch the point, Carter, propolis might qualify as a cell-food, but it should more properly be termed 'ammunition' because it offers elements which assist us cells in fighting infections of all kinds."

"I know all that, Larry."

"Don't ask me to comment if you don't want to hear what I have to say, Carter," he shot back quickly. "I suppose you also know why royal jelly is often called the 'longevity factor.' "

"Yes, I do. It's because. . ."

He interrupted me impatiently. "It's because the Queen bee is *not* conceived genetically superior to any other larva in the hive, but is made royal by her exclusive diet of royal jelly. When the bees recognize that their existing queen is becoming tired, they go to work to produce a new queen. The bees prepare special queen cells, much larger and more spacious than the small cells needed to incubate the tiny larvae destined to be the workers of the hive. The larvae deposited in the queen cells, identical in *every* respect to every other bee larva, are fed royal jelly and very carefully tended. Because there can only be one queen, the first queen larva to emerge immediately destroys the old queen and all the still-sleeping queen larvae.

"After her mating flight, which is the only time she leaves the hive, the Queen settles down to her life's work and fills the brood cells constantly to replenish the population of the hive. The queen feasts on only royal jelly for the whole of her extended lifetime. In nature, a queen bee, whose cells are kept in peak condition by her royal diet, may live a productive life for five or six *years*. In contrast, the Queen's sexless sister bees who are forbidden the royal diet, live for mere weeks before they are worn out and die."

I felt exactly as my own students must feel when I got on a soapbox in class and went over a subject they already knew. "That's very interesting, Larry. Thanks for the lecture."

"You asked. I answered," he responded tartly.

"And I appreciate it. There's a few other supplements I want to check out with you."

"For instance?"

"I found an encapsulized garlic formula that I think is pretty good. Research shows that garlic has spectacular health-promoting properties and I love it. But Bonnie doesn't appreciate the characteristic lingering odor it leaves behind."

"We cells can't tell that garlic is a strong and smelly herb. But we do welcome the elements present in garlic that aid us in our fight to keep your body clean. In fact, garlic helps us normalize blood pressure and reduce cholesterol levels. But if Bonnie doesn't like it and doesn't want you to eat it..."

"No problem. A company called Fountain of Health puts out a nicely formulated product called *Garlic Plus*. This is biologically-active all-organic garlic naturally deodorized with nature's best deodorizer and cleanser, chlorophyll-rich parsley. Garlic Plus also contains cayenne, which the manufacturer says synergistically boosts the action of the garlic."

"Sounds good to me, Carter. The very real benefits of garlic, plus the internal cleansing action of parsley, and cayenne, which is a known potentiating agent. Sometimes you humans do find ways to improve on nature," he answered admiringly. "But what about additives that we can't use and have to defend against? No matter how good the main natural ingredients in a supplement might be, we don't want 'em if they contain alien chemicals, you know."

"Not to worry, you analytical amoeba," I answered affectionately. "The Fountain of Health people agree with you. Not one of their products contains added sodium, sugars, starches, artificial flavors or dyes, or chemical preservatives or laboratory-produced antioxidants."

"I'm relieved, Carter. Believe me, that makes us cells feel a lot better. And when we feel better, so do you."

"I've been conducting a little experiment lately, Larry, just to check out something you said." I smiled to myself. "I wanted to see if I could fool you."

"Don't fool with your immune system defense forces, Professor Carter," he said indignantly. "I'll thank you to remember that I'm a highly-educated sensitized T cell. They don't call me The Terminator for nothing, you know. Without us, you'd be a mass of mucus full of putrifying gunk!"

"Calm down, you microscopic mutant!" I was laughing in spite of myself at his prideful tirade. "Let me explain."

"You'd better," he answered grimly. "And I am *not* a mutant."

"No, of course you're not," I soothed. "We've been so busy with the book that I haven't been able to sit down and eat with the family lately. Bonnie has been going all out preparing good whole cell-foods, but I've been preoccupied and grabbing my meals at odd times. I've been compensating for my nutritional lapses by taking more supplements."

"I haven't noticed a lack of any particular nutrients lately, Carter." He sounded puzzled. "You must be eating right."

"I'm glad to hear you say that, Larry. If they fooled you, the *Fiber Plus* and *Beta-Carotene Plus* supplements from Fountain of Health must be okay."

"Well," he mused aloud, "I can tell that you've stepped up your fiber intake. That's very important to our purposes, Carter. In the U.S., the average daily intake of fiber is around 4 grams. You should take in close to 30 grams of fiber every day. Your scientists have discovered that in countries where fiber intake is high, cancers of the colon are virtually nonexistent. I've been noticing that the constituents of all seven major fiber groups have been available to us cells recently."

"I know that, Larry. *Fiber Plus* contains true organic fiber from the major fiber groups, plus the important minerals that science says the body loses at an accelerated rate when the digestive and intestinal tracts are stimulated by adequate fiber and working at top efficiency."

"The body does lose calcium, magnesium, and zinc when additional fiber is added to the diet. But I haven't noticed any deficiencies, Carter."

"Of course not. The *'plus'* in Fiber Plus is the addition of precisely these minerals," I explained.

"Very good. It looks like these Fountain of Health people

know what they're about. Do they prepare other organic supplements, too?"

"You bet. They have a complete range of naturally-formulated products, like *Beta-Carotene Plus.* This one is produced from organically grown Dunaliella Kona from Kailua-Kona, Hawaii. This stuff is very special. Dunaliella Kona offers a rich abundance of beta-carotene, more than any other vegetable source, including carrots. You'll also appreciate the fact that the beta-carotene is extracted without chemicals and is stabilized with the natural antioxidants, vitamins A and E."

"You're right. I do appreciate that. And I appreciate the fact that beta-carotene acts to destroy the layer of mucus surrounding a cancer cell. That makes our job easier. Beta-carotene helps us develop strong protection against cancers of the lungs and bronchia, and colorectal cancers as well. Your medical scientists say that reductions in the incidence of lung cancer when beta-carotene is included in the daily diet can amount to 80 percent. And the chance of contracting colon cancer is reduced by 55 percent for those who take beta-carotene."

"Wow!" I said, suitably impressed with his ready recall of material I had researched months ago. "Very important statistics, Larry."

"You bet they are, Carter. What other products have you discovered to make my job easier?"

"There's *Calcium Plus.* This supplement offers organic calcium, plus phosphorus and magnesium, with no harmful fillers or chemical additives."

"Sounds good, Carter. Those are the very elements we need to build and maintain strong bones and teeth and protect you from the brittle bones of osteoporosis or the soft spongy bones of osteomalacia. And remember, too, that rebounding strengthens bone density. I'd say you are well protected."

"That's good news! How do you feel about lactobacillus acidophilus, Larry? Fountain of Health also offers *L-Acidophilus*

Plus."

"We like that friendly bacteria, Carter. It's immensely helpful to our body. Lactobacillus acidophilus is vital to the entire gastro-intestinal system. It controls yeast organisms, fights infections, and eliminates chronic diarrhea. Do you know that antibiotics wipe out entire colonies of this helpful bacteria, thereby weakening your defense forces by overworking us?"

"I did know that, Larry."

"I'm curious, Carter. I must have been off-duty when you went shopping for everything we've been writing about in our book. Did you find it all in a cell-food store?"

"What you like to call cell-food stores, we call health-food stores, Larry. And don't pretend you don't know better, you aggravating little amoeba. And, yes, I found most of the health-building products we've been talking about in that big health food store here in the great state of Washington where we live. Most, but not all, that is."

"If the health-food store doesn't have what they're looking for, how will our readers find what they need? I foresee a problem here," he said sternly. "I distinctly remember that it was *your* job to search out the best of everything, Carter. What have you got to say for yourself, you meaty monolith?"

"Hold on, Larry. I object to your lack of faith in me. I know we have an obligation to our readers. You should know that I wouldn't leave them out on a limb. I've been having a lot of the good stuff we've been talking about shipped to us via United Parcel Service. Our readers can do the same thing. In fact, this seems like a good place to put in the name and address of New Dimensions Distributors. They have been taking good care of us and I know they'll do right by our readers, too. The very knowledgeable people at New Dimensions make it easy to shop by mail or phone."

"And they handle *everything*, Carter? Even the water purifiers and the Rebound exercisers?"

"Everything, Larry."

"Do they really have all the supplements we just reviewed, Carter? And the bee pollen, Carter. don't forget the bee pollen."

"Everything, Larry."

"Stop blathering and do it then, Carter."

"Right," I agreed. "But you're the one blathering on." So, dear reader, as Larry instructed, I obediently typed in:

New Dimensions Distributors
16548 E. Laser Drive, #A-7
Fountain Hills, Arizona 85268
Call: 1-800-624-7114 Toll-Free Nationwide
In Arizona (602), Call: 1-837-8322

"Now we have that important information in, I think we're ready to close up shop for the night, little buddy. I appreciate all your input on these supplements, but this has been a very long session."

"I do believe we've about covered everything, Carter. Incidentally, the next 36 hours are going to be very full for me. I've been meaning to give you some advance notice. . ."

"Excuse me, Larry. I just can't concentrate any longer." I covered my mouth and yawned hugely as I clicked off the word processor. I stood and stretched, trying to work out the kinks that had developed while I sat hunched over the machine.

"But, Carter, you need to know. . ."

"Give it a rest, Larry. We'll pick up tomorrow where we left off, okay?"

"Whatever you say *Professor.*" If he had been human, he would have sighed in exasperation.

I was too tired to notice that he called me 'Professor,' a sure sign he was miffed. I yawned again as I shuffled wearily off to bed.

CHAPTER 17

THANKS FOR THE MEMORIES

"Larry. Larry? Where *are* you? Speak to me, oh mighty molecule."

"Can't you call Larry quietly, dear?" Bonnie mumbled as she peered at me with sleepy eyes. "It's almost midnight."

"Under normal circumstances, I can. I've been thinking about him for the past few days, but I haven't had a response."

"Well, please go in the front room and yell for him, if you must. Anything so I can get some sleep."

Her request was not unreasonable. I guess I had been unbearable the past few days. I had delivered my manuscript. . . our manuscript, Larry's and mine. . . to a publishing company in Arizona and presented it to them. They loved it! The publisher told me it was refreshing to find a "hero" who could actually "talk to himself" without sounding crazy. The editor assigned to helping us smooth out the rough edges simply fell in love with Larry. As she really got into the book, she confided to me that she almost felt as if she should "apologize" to Larry whenever she ate something that couldn't qualify as a good cell-food.

Publishing contracts had been signed. I had approved the

231

minor changes our editor suggested during several story conferences. All but the last two chapters of the manuscript had been turned over to the typesetter. I felt terrific! I just knew that all the cells of my entire lymphatic army were celebrating much as our soldiers did on V-Day, but I had a nagging feeling that something was wrong. Thinking back, I couldn't remember Larry making any comments at all during the negotiations with the publisher. I guess I assumed that, because he had no negative reaction, he approved. I mean, getting our book published was his whole purpose, wasn't it? The last thing the publisher had said to me was, "Al, get those last chapters in to us just as soon as you and Larry can get it together so we can go to press with the book."

"It's as good as done," I answered, feeling sure that I was speaking for both Larry and myself. I was tingling all over on the way back home from Phoenix. I remember thinking, 'This must be the way champagne feels just before somebody pops the cork!' I felt I was ready to pop any second.

Bonnie had picked me up at the Sea-Tac Airport near Seattle, commenting in her gentle way that I was radiating success.

"Of course, dear," I remember answering. "Haven't you heard that everyone has at least one book in them?"

"Yes. But you didn't know you had it in you until Larry showed up," she pointed out.

All that had transpired over forty-eight hours ago. Fifty-one and one-half hours ago, to be exact. Bonnie is asleep again. I'm sitting here in front of the word processor waiting. And waiting.

"I'm waiting, Larry. Nothing is happening, Larry. A book isn't finished until the last chapter is written, Larry. I need you Larry. The publisher can't go to press until we send him the final pages. You know that, don't you, Larry?

"Speak to me, Larry. Let your presence be known by attacking a nerve. Cause a sharp pain in my back, my eye, my foot, anywhere. We're so close to accomplishing your objective. I need your help right now!

"Ouch!" I sat up straight. "Ouch!" I said even louder. "One jab will do, you lily-livered lympho! Where have you been hiding out anyway? Oooo, that hurts. Stop it! Where are you? My leg or my back? They both hurt at the same time. You're full of tricks, aren't you? Look, asking you to signal me with pain wasn't such a good idea. Why don't you migrate to the semi-circular canals of my inner ear, or perhaps the stirrup so you can talk to me? I'll wait. No, better yet, I'll rebound to speed up my lymphatic circulation. That will help you get there faster."

I hopped up on The Rebound and began to jog in place vigorously. "This is really strange, Larry. I feel you buzzing in my head, but I can't make out what you're trying to say. In fact, I'm getting a buzzing in both ears. Where are you? Right or left?"

"Can you hear me, sir?"

"Nod your head, if you understand me, Professor Carter."

"Hey! Not so loud. Of course, I understand you. How can you be in two places at once? What's with you? You act as if you've never communicated with me before."

My right ear buzzed, "I haven't."

My left ear buzzed, "Neither have I."

"Wait!" It was beginning to make sense. "Larry. . . you haven't. . . Yes, you have. I've got it. You've divided, haven't you? That's the only possible explanation. There are two of you now. One in each ear. Am I right?"

"Yes. I . . . we . . . have. It happens to every cell that survives long enough." I heard the words distinctly in my left ear.

I sensed more than heard in my right ear, "I really don't know how to respond, oh Great Body. Your slightest thought is my command. My job is to listen and obey; to protect unto death; to search out and destroy all foreign enemies. . ."

"You are the sons of Larry, aren't you?"

"If you say so, oh Great One," came the timid response in

my right ear.

"Not really," the voice in my left ear answered quickly. "Not the same way humans have sons and daughters, Professor Carter. You see, when the T-Cell you called 'Larry' divided, our mitosis lasted about thirty hours. When our DNA started to duplicate, all our energy went into replication. There was no way to communicate with you until the entire replication had taken place. It took all of the energy we could squeeze from our mitochondria to produce the enzymes necessary to sustain life. It's a jungle in here, you know."

"There are two of you now," I said with delight as I began to realize what had taken place. "What shall I call you?"

"Anything that pleases you, Your Greatness." The tiny sound came from deep inside my head on the right.

"We don't go by human names in here, Professor," corrected the voice on the left. "It isn't necessary to call us out individually, you know. In fact, it isn't necessary to call us at all. We know our jobs. Your body is safe with us."

"Wait a minute" I objected. "I know you know your responsibilities inside me, but what about the book Larry and I have been working on? Don't you think that's important?"

"Yes, Great One," the voice on the right said deferentially. "Anything important to you is important to us. We will do whatever you desire."

Sounding more and more like Larry, the voice on the left buzzed, "Professor, are you aware of how dangerous it is for us to be communicating with you by producing these vibrations.?"

"Personal danger is of no concern to us, sir," the voice on the right buzzed primly.

"What danger are you talking about?" I asked.

"Larry was lucky, Professor Carter. He was functioning beyond the programming of a Cytotoxic T-Lymphocyte by managing to communicate with you directly. According to the bylaws of the body, that is an illegal act. Punishment is immediate destruction by ingestion. I really don't know how he got away with it. My life is in jeopardy right now because I am communicating with you in an un-lymphocyte-like manner. If I don't function exactly as I should, I could be identified as a mutant cell. That means sure death."

"You obviously know how to communicate with me," I said reasonably. "You're doing it right now."

"Of course. All the knowledge contained in Larry's DNA was duplicated during replication. But that doesn't mean I have to use it. Or, if I do communicate with you directly, I don't have to like it. And now there are two of us with the knowledge."

All I need is the closing chapter of the book Larry and I are writing. Is that asking too much?"

"It might indeed be asking too much."

I was getting desperate. "Look," I said sternly, "you owe that much to Larry *and* to me. If it *were* not for both of us, you wouldn't exist right now."

After a lengthy pause, the answer came. "You are correct, Professor Carter. And since you put it that way, I will help. But only to approve or disapprove. You write. If you get something wrong, I'll let you know."

"How will I know?"

"You'll know."

"Thank you," I said formally, longing for Larry himself and the camaraderie we had established over the many months we had worked together. I wasn't quite sure how this arrangement was going to work out. Feeling a little lonely, I decided to begin by making an outline of the most important things I had learned from Larry.

I.   *Cancer Is A Misnomer*

The word 'cancer' is Latin for crab. Several hundred years ago, long before medical doctors discovered that all types of cancer arise as a result of the mutation of the body cells themselves, the physicians of the day thought that cancer resembled a crab.

II. *Cancer Is Not A Disease*

The medical definition of disease is: 'Something foreign to the body which attacks it.' Cancer does not fit that definition. All cancers are produced by the body itself. Cancer occurs when mutant cells are allowed to proliferate unchecked.

III. *Nothing 'Causes' Cancer. An Inefficient Immune System Permits Cancer to Develop.*

The only way mutant cells can progress into cancerous cells is if the immune system fails to identify them as 'traitors.' Cancer develops only when the immune system is too weak, is improperly nourished, is overworked and/or exhausted from defending against too many foreign substances, or when all of the above factors are combined.

IV. *In Order To Qualify As A Cancer Cell, Two Mutations Must Occur*

There are certain genes in every cell which control the growth and reproduction of that cell. Mutations must occur in both growth and reproductive genes before a cell is capable of developing into a cancerous cell.

V. *Immune System Cells Can Be Strengthened Or Weakened*

Every cell in the body has the ability to become stronger or weaker in response to internal environmental factors. Nutrition and exercise programs undertaken by an individual directly affect the internal environment of the cells of the body, either positively or negatively. Every cell, including the lymphocytes of the immune system, grow stronger (or weaker) in response to the nutrients we eat (or don't eat), the exercise we take (or don't take), and the purity (or pollution) of the water we drink.

I read over what I had typed with a critical eye. I felt I had pretty well summarized the pertinent points Larry had been hammering home. With all the puzzle pieces in front of me, the answer to cancer seemed almost too ridiculously simple.

I sat back and said aloud, "How am I doing so far, Sons of Larry?"

Words of praise buzzed promptly in my right ear. "You are so wise, oh Great Body." If this particular Son of Larry was going to continue giving me unqualified approval and what seemed uncomfortably like "worship," he wasn't going to be much help at all.

Almost simultaneously, I felt a warm tingling sensation at the base of my skull. I decided that meant the other Son of Larry approved, but I couldn't help wishing fervently for one of Larry's sarcastic comments. What Larry had been teaching all along, I realized, was what each of us must do to keep the cells of our immune system healthy. It seemed time to gather all I had learned from his preaching under some sort of an umbrella. After he worked so hard to bring the book this far along, I sure didn't want to let him down at the end.

Larry himself would probably say, "Get on with it, Carter." I chuckled a little to myself and "got on with it."

CHAPTER 18

THE HEALTHY CELL CONCEPT

While I was trying to figure out how to present an all-encompassing overview of Larry's teaching, I sat quietly with my hands on the keys. Old habits die hard, especially happy ones. I was unconsciously waiting for Larry to crackle in my ear. Suddenly, the perfect title was impressed upon my mind somehow. I thought - no, *hoped* - that the impression was coming to me from a Son of Larry. I obediently backed up and headed this concluding chapter:

The Healthy Cell Concept

The Body

All 75 trillion cells which make up the body live together and interact perfectly in a complex social order. Cells are organized into different functional structures or "families," known as blood cells (red and white), bones, organs, and connective tissue. Each family of cells contributes its share to insure the correct maintenance of homeostatic conditions in the internal environment. As long as healthy conditions are maintained, all families of cells will continue to live and function properly. Thus, each cell contributes its share to maintain homeostasis, and each cell benefits.

This reciprocal interplay of all cells in effect runs the body "on automatic." Continuous automaticity will continue indefinitely until and unless one or more of the functional systems families of cells loses the ability to bear its share of the load. If this happens, all the cells of the body suffer. Moderate dysfunction leads to illness, but extreme dysfunction can progress unto death.

If we humans understand this and provide what our cells need, we won't have to worry about dying of cancer. Larry had very effectively drummed that into me. I remembered, too, that he had proven himself correct every time by guiding me to authoritative scientific reference material. Because there are at least four ways we humans can help our immune system defense forces do their job more efficiently, *The Healthy Cell Concept* can be divided into four integral and equally important parts.

I. *Cell Food*

All cells need the proper nutrients to keep them healthy. Simply stated, cell food is the kind of food the cells themselves would select if they had the ability to do the grocery shopping. A cell's grocery cart would be full of whole foods from which they can extract (or synthesize) the elements they need to keep the body functioning at top efficiency. And, given the choice, a cell on a shopping expedition would never select any manufactured or processed food product containing elements foreign to the body.

II. *Cell Environment*

All cells depend on extracellular fluid for transport of oxygen and nutrients *in*, and the carrying of waste byproducts *out*. This fluid is water. Extracellular fluid is also the universal catalyst of all chemical activity inside the cells. Lymphocytes depend on lymph fluid (extracellular water) for transport. These essential cells of the immune system travel waterways to get from one part of the body to another. Pure water is a basic necessity for the healthy functioning of the immune system, and the healthy functioning of the entire body.

III. *Cell Exercise*

In close analysis, it appears that all the usual forms of exercise contribute mainly to the self-gratification of the individual. In our preoccupation with body-image, we have given nary a thought to the health of the 75 trillion cells of the body. Too-strenuous exercise actually destroys millions of cells. Double-trouble. We not only lose the use of the cells which have died, but the lymphocytes are unnecessarily overloaded. It is their responsibility to cleanse the body of the dead cells. And when they're scooting around busily doing just that, other more important work is neglected.

Good cell exercise provides cellular resistance, but without approaching the rupture threshold of the cells. Good cell exercise increases circulation of the blood and lymph, and stimulates respiratory function, thereby increasing oxygen delivery to every cell. Admittedly, any type of exercise is better than no exercise at all. But only rebound exercise meets or exceeds all criteria for an ideal cell exercise.

IV. *Cell Communication*

Is it possible that Jesus Christ was able to heal the sick and raise Lazareth from the dead simply because he spoke a universal language understood by all elements of His creation? Will we ever learn?

We seldom eavesdrop on them, but cells communicate constantly with one another. We only pay attention when cellular communication makes us feel hungry, sleepy, or hurt. We have the ability to communicate instantaneously with our cells. In fact, we do it all the time without thinking much about it. Our cells are perfectly attuned to our every thought. The ability of cells to communicate is greater and faster than the puny human's. Instead of expecting cells to communicate as we do, we should learn their language. When we learn to properly interpret the language of the cells of our own body, we will not only have the answer to cancer, but to all other human frailties as well.

I leaned back and read over the presentation so far. The Healthy Cell Concept formed into a clear-cut picture in my mind, with Larry, the ultimate spokesman for healthy cells everywhere, at center. Idly, I sketched it out. Yes, I thought with satisfaction, Larry would approve. This will make it easier for humans to visualize the four factors necessary to a healthy immune system. Here it is:

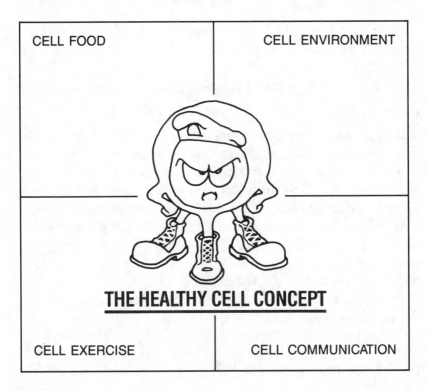

CELL FOOD	CELL ENVIRONMENT
THE HEALTHY CELL CONCEPT	
CELL EXERCISE	CELL COMMUNICATION

I was mentally congratulating myself when I heard it:

"Professor, under the possiblity of immediate destruction, I will break my silence to ask a very important question. If everything you say in this book is true, and I agree that it is, surely you have examples of humans who have lived by the simple rules of The Healthy Cell Concept and thereby received the blessings of health of which you write?"

I felt like jumping up from my chair and cheering! I was afraid to scare him away, so I answered mildly instead. "Yes, Son of Larry. I'll tell you about some of them."

"Don't tell me, Professor. I know what you know. Tell your reader. They're the ones who need to hear about some faith-promoting experiences. Why don't you lead off with David of Oregon? His story is simple, sweet, and verifiable."

"Good idea."

"I know."

"You sound just like Larry," I said, trying not to sound as delighted as I was.

"I know."

Without further words, I began typing:

David Salisbury. Astoria, Oregon

David was twenty-nine years old and appeared to be in relatively good health when he noticed a knot about the size of a softball deep in the left side of his abdomen. Because he felt all right and had no reason to think otherwise, he told himself it was the result of the big dinner he had eaten a few days before. Not wanting to worry his wife, Shari, he kept the discovery to himself for several days. But the lump didn't go away, and finally he confided in her. They decided together that it must be an impacted colon.

A month after David noticed the knot, the young couple decided they should seek professional advice. They visited their chiropractor, Dean Simmons, D.C., in Tacoma, Washington. Dr. Simmons said, "I'm quite sure this isn't an impacted colon, David. You'd better have it checked by a medical doctor."

After returning to Astoria, David had to wait another two and one-half weeks before he could get in to see a medical doctor. This doctor promptly chastised him for waiting two months after the discovery of the lump before getting medical advice.

David explains, "What I thought was going to be a brief examination turned into a day-long ordeal of tests and x-rays. I knew then that the doctors were more than a little concerned about my condition. They told me there was a good chance that my lump was a lymphoma. They scheduled a biopsy for me."

On April 24th, David Salisbury was wheeled into surgery at Columbia Memorial Hospital for a procedure called a *mediastinoscopy,* a method of securing tissue samples for microscopic diagnosis, to confirm the results of his physical exam the day before.

The initial report read in part: ". . . On abdominal examination, there is a firm tender mass about the size of a volley ball in the left upper quadrant." The pathologist's report on the two excised tissue specimens read in part: ". . . malignant lymphoma, nodular type."

David was immediately referred to a cancer specialist in Portland, Oregon. He had to wait three weeks and received a prescription for chemotherapy on his second visit. He was also told his cancer had advanced to Stage III. With guarded optimism, the cancer specialist said, "Your attitude is good. Physically, you seem to be feeling remarkably well considering that large load of cancer you're carrying around."

"Isn't it true that most humans would give up after hearing that?" This query came from the Son of Larry in my left ear.

"Most would, but not David," I answered and continued typing. David was determined to find out if there was an alternative to the chemotherapy and surgery that was surely ahead of him.

David explains, "We had seen a rebounder before, but

now we really had a reason to be interested. We bought a rebounder, along with a good supply of herbs and distilled water. I immediately went into training."

"That's great!" enthused the Son of Larry. "Had you told him about The Healthy Cell Concept, Professor?"

"No. I didn't know David at that time. As a matter of fact, I didn't know about The Healthy Cell Concept back then either."

"Tell our readers what David did, Professor."

He said 'our readers,' I noted with satisfaction, hoping he was evolving into a full-fledged 'Larry' on his own. "We'll let David tell it himself. He lived it."

David continued, "I went on a ten-day colon and body cleansing diet. I eliminated red meat, bleached flour, sugar, and dairy products from my diet. I ate fresh fruits and vegetables. I also ate lots of whole grains, including homemade whole wheat bread, and I drank lots of pure water. My meat intake was limited to poultry or light fish two to three times per week. In addition to this healthy diet, I also bounced for thirty to sixty minutes per day on the rebounder."

"That got his lymphatic system flowing," Son of Larry put in.

"That's just what David said," I agreed. "Not only that, but this remarkable man had faith in his Creator and asked his friends to pray for him."

"Cellular communication," I heard distinctly.

"Communication both directions." I reminded him.

"Of course," declared Son of Larry excitedly. "I was just acknowledging that David employed every step of the Healthy Cell Concept as we taught you. Cell food, cell exercise, cell environment, and cell communication. I can't wait. Type in what happened next, Professor."

David has a letter from Gary M. Boelling, M.D. dated September 23rd, 1980, which states, "Enclosed is a copy of the x-ray report from your x-ray taken the 22nd of September. As you can see, the radiologist sees no evidence of tumor remaining."

"Ya Hoo!" I felt, more than heard. "Hurray for our side!" I was smiling as I asked, "Did you have any doubts?"

"Certainly not," he snapped. "We cells see such victories every day. But maybe this story will get through the thick craniums of some of the humans running your world. Has there been any recurrence of David's cancerous condition?"

"Nope," I replied. "I have copies of the letters David's doctor sent him reporting the results of his annual checkups for the following five years. Shall I give you more examples of people who overcame cancer?"

"I don't need more examples, Professor. That would be like asking a police officer if he wanted to see reports of additional arrests. Or like asking a baker if he needed a recipe for making his favorite bread."

"You're right, of course. I really didn't think of it that way. I was thinking that maybe the readers. . ."

"Professor," he cut in, "If our readers don't understand The Healthy Cell Concept by now, it's too late."

"I guess you're right," I acknowledged.

"Consider all the humans that the cancer specialists claim to have cured. Those humans have been through surgery, chemotherapy, even radiation. I remind you that all those procedures kill healthy cells, as well as malignant ones. These patients leave the hospital praising the talents of their doctors and the hospital staff. Many times, for good reason. They are congratulated and assured they are among those who have survived cancer. But who has the responsibility of keeping them alive and well for the rest of their lives?"

"It's yours."

"You are right. And don't you forget it."

"I won't."

"I know."

"Excuse me, Professor Carter," the tiny voice sounded in my left ear. "I'm more concerned about what you personally are going to do about the information in this book. It was brought to your attention so that our jobs would be made easier."

"I'm sorry, " I said. "I forgot for a moment that there were two of you."

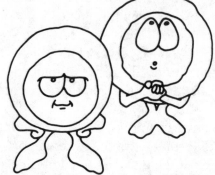

"Actually, there are trillions of us, Oh Great Body. We depend on you for our very sustenance. Please be benevolent and grant us our needs."

"That is a request beneficial to all. I have already promised to do everything in my power to continue living The Healthy Cell Concept."

"Oh, thank you, Great Body, for being so considerate. May you live forever."

"Please, not that," I answered fervently. "I just ask to be healthy until I die."

"We know."

It's all really simple, I thought. I was satisfied as I tapped out:

The End

"Wait, Professor," the Son of Larry buzzed in my left ear. "That's not quite correct. It may confuse our readers. Just learning about The Healthy Cell concept isn't enough. It's up to each human to provide for the cells of their bodies. They must practice what we cells preach. Let us close our book:

The Beginning of the Rest of Your Life"

Bibliography

Chapter 1

DiPolo, R and Beauge, L: The Calcium Pump and Sodium-Calcium Exchange in Squid Axons. Annu Rev Physiol., 45:313, 1983.

Hodgkin, AL, and Huxley, AF: Quantitative Description of Membrane Current and Its Application to Conduction and Excitation in Nerve. J Physiol, London: 117:500, 1952.

Taubes, G: An Electrifying Possibility. Discover Magazine, April 1986.

Chapter 2

Antoniades, HN, and Owen, AJ: Growth Factors and Regulation of Cell Growth. Annu Rev Med, 33:445, 1982.

Bryant, PJ and Simpson, P: Intrinsic and Extrinsic Control of Growth in Developing Organs. Q Rev Biol, 59:387, 1984.

Davidson, R: Somatic Cell Genetics. New York: Van Nostrand Reinhold, 1984.

Guyton, AC: Text Book of Medical Physiology. Philadelphia: WB Saunders Co 1986.

Hall, A: Oncogenes-Implications for Human Cancer: A Review. J R Soc Med, 77:410, 1984.

Horton, JD (ed): Development and Differentation of Vertebrates. New York: Elsevier/North Holland, 1980.

Pablo, CO, and Sauer, RT: Protein-DNA Recognition. Annu Rev Biochem 53:293, 1984.

Chapter 3

Atkins, MD, RZ Dr. Atkins' Nutrition Breakthrough. New York: William Morrow and Co, Inc 1981.

Gadebusch, HJ (ed): Phagocytosis and Cellular Immunity. West Palm Beach, FL: CRC Press, 1979.

Quastel, MR (ed): Cell Biology and Immunology of Leukocyte Function. New York: Academic Press, 1979.

Chapter 4

Fudenberg, HH and Smith, CL (eds): The Lymphocyte in Health and Disease. New York: Grune and Stratton, 1979.

Getenby, PA, et al: T-Cells, T-Cell Subsets and Immune Regulation. Aust N Z J Med, 14:89, 1984.

Guyton, AC: Text Book of Medical Physiology. Philadelphia: WB Saunders Co, 1986.

Kendall, MD: Have We Underestimated the Importance of the Thymus in Man? Experientia, 40:1181, 1984.

Sercarz, EE and Cunningham, AJ (eds): Strategies of Immune Regulation. New York: Academic Press, 1979.

Chapter 5

Fischer, WL: How to Fight Cancer and Win. Canfield, Ohio: Fischer Publishing

Guyton, AC: Text Book of Medical Physiology. Philadelphia: WB Saunders Co, 1986.

Holleb, AI, MD, (ed): The American Cancer Society Cancer Book. Garden City, New York: Doubleday and Co, 1986.

McCally, M: Hypodynamics and Hypogravics: The Physiology of Inactivity and Weightlessness. New York: Academic Press, 1969.

Sandler, H and Winter, DL: Physiological Responses of Women to Simulated Weightlessness. Springfield, VA: National Technical Information Service, 1978.

Chapter 6

The Congressional Quarterly. April, 1986.

Statistical Abstract: US Dept of Commerce, 1987.

US Budget in Brief: Executive Office of the President, 1987.

Chapter 7

Devita, BT: Cancer Treatment. US Department of Health and Human Services.

Guyton, AC: Text Book of Medical Physiology. Philadelphia: WB Saunders Co, 1986.

Laws, PW: X-Rays - More Harm than Good? Emmaus, PA: Rodale, 1977.

Morra, M and Potts, A: Choices, Realistic Alternatives in Cancer Treatment. New York: Avon Books, 1980.

Null, G and Steinman, L: A Billion Dollar Boondoggle. New York: Penthouse, 1985.

Salsbury, KH and Johnson, EL: Indispensable Cancer Handbook. New York: Seaview Books, 1981.

Smedley, H, Sikora, K and Stepney, R: Cancer, What It Is and How It's Treated. Oxford, Great Britain: Basil Blackwell Ltd, 1985.

Washington Post, Washington DC: 1977.

Winter, R: Cancer Causing Agents. New York: Crown Publishers Inc, 1979.

Chapter 8

Holleb, AI, MD (ed): The American Cancer Society Cancer Book. Garden City, New York: Doubleday and Co, 1986.

Smedley, H, Sikora, K and Stephney, R: Cancer, What It Is and How It's Treated. Oxford, Great Britian: Basil Blackwell Ltd, 1985.

Winter, R: Cancer Causing Agents. New York: Crown Publishers Inc, 1979.

Chapter 9

Atkins, MD, RZ: Dr. Atkins' Nutrition Breakthrough. New York: William Morrow and Co, 1981.

Baram, P, et al (eds): Immunologic Tolerance and Macrophage Function. Holland: Elsevier/North, 1979.

Guyton, AC: Text Book of Medical Physiology. Philadelphia: WB Saunders Co, 1986.

Ham, AW, et al: Blood Cell Formation and the Cellular Basis of Immune Responses. Philidelphia: JB Lippincott Co, 1979.

Lancki, EW, et al: Cell Surface Structures Involved in T-Cell Activation. Immunol. Rev, 81:65 1984.

Chapter 10

Atkins, MD, RZ: Dr. Atkins' Nutrition Breakthrough. New York: William Morrow and Co, 1981.

Gerson, M: A Cancer Therapy - Results of Fifty Cases. Delmar, CA: Totality Books, 1977.

Guyton, AC: Text Book of Medical Physiology. Philadelphia: WB Saunders Co, 1986.

Smedley, H, Sikora, K and Stepney, R: Cancer, What It Is and How It's Treated. Oxford, Great Britain: Basil Blackwell Ltd, 1985.

Chapter 11

Atkins, MD, RZ: Dr. Atkins' Nutrition Breakthrough. New York: William Morrow and Co, 1981.

Fischer, WL: How to Fight Cancer and Win. Canfield, Ohio: Fischer Publishing Corporation, 1987.

Guyton, AC: Text Book of Medical Physiology. Philadelphia: WB Saunders Co, 1986.

Robinson, CH: Fundamentals in Normal Nutrition. New York: MacMillian, 1973.

Svacha, AJ, Wesson, NC and Waslein, CI: Effect of Egg Intake and Tobacco Smoking on Serum Cholesterol. Fed Proc 33:690, 1974.

Chapter 12

Biesel, ND, WR: Nutrient Effects on Immunologic Functions. Journal American Medical Association, January 1981.

Burack, ND, WR: Lies and Statistics. Medical World News, August 1979.

Passwater, PhD, R: Cancer and Its Nutritional Therapies. New Canaan, Conn: Keats Pub, 1978.

Pfeiffer, CC: Mental and Elemental Nutrients. New Canaan: Keats Publishing Inc, 1975.

Svacha, AJ, Wesson, NC, and Waslein, CI: Effect of Egg Intake and Tobacco Smoking on Serum Cholesterol. Fed Proc, 33:690, 1974.

Chapter 13

Carter, AE: The Miracles of Rebound Exercise. Edmonds, WA: The National Institute of Reboundology and Health, 1979.

Guyton, AC: Text Book of Medical Physiology. Philadelphia: WB Saunders Co, 1986.

Chapter 14

Alabaster, MD, O: What You Can Do To Prevent Cancer. New York: Simon and Schuster, 1985.

Bragg, ND, PhD, PC: The Shocking Truth About Water. Santa Barbara, CA: Health Science.

Chen,PS: Inorganic, Organic and Biological Chemistry. New York: Harper and Rowe, 1979.

Gotzsche, AL: The Fluoride Question. Briercliff Manor, New York: Stein and Day, 1975.

Guyton, AC: Text Book of Medical Physiology. Philadelphia: WB Saunders Co, 1986.

Salsbury, KH and Johnson, EL: Indispensable Cancer Hand-book, New York: Seaview Books, 1981.

Yiamouyiannis, PhD, John: Fluoride: The Aging Factor. Delaware, Ohio: Health Action Press, 1983.

Chapter 15

Guyton, AC: Text Book of Medical Physiology. Philadelphia: WB Saunders Co, 1986.

Hales, A: Mind Over Matter - Facts about Psycho-Immunity. Science Digest Magazine. New York: The Hearst Corp, November 1981.

Korombokis, L: Faith Healers in the Laboratory. Science Digest. New York: The Hearst Corp, May 1982.

Nolen, WA: The Woman Said, "No," to Cancer. Science Digest. December 1982. Excerpted from A Surgeons Hand Book of Hope. Coward, McCann, and Geoghegan 1980.

Star, D: Interspecies Communication. Omni Magazine, New York: Omni Pub, December 1986.

Chapter 16

Erasmus, Udo: Fats & Oils. Vancouver, BC, Canada: Alive Press 1986.

Ioyrish, Naum: Bees and People. Moscow, USSR: MIR Publishers, 1977.

Robinson, MD, William: Journal of the National Cancer Institute. Oct 1948, 119-123.

Wade, Carson: Bee Pollen & Your Health, New Canaan, Connecticut: Keats Publishing, Inc, 1978.

Diet, Nutrition & Cancer Prevention. US Dept Health & Human Services, 1984.

Encyclopedia of Common Diseases. Emmaus, PA: Rodale Press, 1976.

The Hive & The Honey Bee. Hamilton, Illinois: Dadant & Sons, 1975.

World's Only Perfect Food. Scottsdale, Arizona: CC Pollen Company, 1984.